WELI

Practical and Spiritual Solutions for Busy People

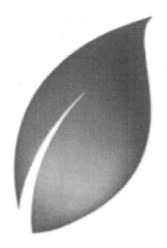

Pamela Maldonado, M.Ed.

Master Christian Life Coach

with

Leelo Bush, Ph.D.

WELLNESS: Practical and Spiritual Solutions for Busy People

Copyright © 2014 by Pamela Maldonado

Published by: Pamela Maldonado

ISBN: 978-0-9913816-0-9

About the Authors

Pamela Maldonado, M.Ed., is a 28-year fitness and nutrition educator and Master Christian Life Coach who specializes in Wellness. Healthy living is second nature for Pam who has made it her life's goal. As a long-time veteran in the field of health and wellness, Pam is especially passionate about helping others achieve their nutritional, exercise, and weight control goals. She also enjoys helping people in other areas of their lives such as relationships, career, and life transition coaching.

"With God, anything is possible!

You just have to trust, believe and get to work!"

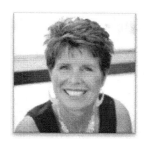 Pam is a sports enthusiast who was a key player for Redwood Falls High School girls' basketball team which won the first Minnesota Girls' State High School Championship in 1976! That was the beginning of her sports career. She later went on to play volleyball and basketball at St. Cloud State University.

Pam holds a Master's in Education degree in curriculum and instruction from the College of St. Scholastica as well as Bachelor of Science degrees from St. Cloud State University in Health Education and Physical Education.

She grew up on a Minnesota dairy farm surrounded by the love of a wonderful, hard- working family. The unshakable faith in God that her parents displayed in their daily lives was the rock that her faith has been modeled after.

Pam lives in southern Minnesota with Efren, her supportive and inspirational husband, and has a grown daughter and son. In her free time, Pam pours herself into her other passion, her two-year-old horse, Sierra.

Leelo Bush, Ph.D., "America's Doctor of Joy," is known globally for her life-transforming personal and professional development and certification programs and books. The heartbeat of her work is her faith in and reverential love of her Savior, Jesus Christ.

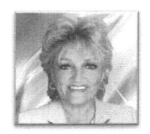

Dr. Bush is a visionary, industry-leading author of the *Christian Coach Handbook: Essential Guide to Spirit Led Coaching and Business Success*, the Christian coaching manifesto that led to the transformation of Christian coaching from use of psychology as its foundation to a true, Spirit-led, Biblical foundation, thereby creating *Christian Coaching 2.0*.

She is president and founder of Beautiful Life International (BLI), LLC, and has authored numerous training and certification programs offered at BLI and the Professional Christian Coaching and Counseling Academy (PCCCA): *Certified Christian Life Coach, Master Christian Life Coach, Joy Restoration©/Christian Grief Coach, Stress Relief Coach©, 7-Step Happiness by Choice Method©, Certified Christian Counselor and Spirit-Led Marketing©.*

Dr. Bush has a Ph.D. and Master's Degree in Christian Counseling from Newburgh Seminary and Bible College as well as Bachelor of Arts degree from Ohio State University in Political Science and English. Among her early mentors have been the late John W. Galbreath, philanthropist, developer, franchise-owner of Pittsburgh Pirates, Kentucky Derby winning thoroughbred breeder and Joe Taylor, a veteran Washington Press Corp Journalist. A lifelong health and fitness proponent, she is also certified in essential oils and business from dōTERRA University.

Leelo Bush is married to Evan Bush, MCLC and has one adult daughter. They reside in southwest Florida and enjoy boating on the Gulf of Mexico, the arts and culinary adventures.

Dedication

To My God, My All . . .

My words do no justice to You. All I can say is thank You for loving me, for Your grace, and for using me as Your servant. All I have in life is because of You. I give You all my thanks and praise!

Living with abundant health and wellness is the best way to glorify God through the miraculous body, mind, and Spirit He has given us!

Acknowledgements

Dr. Bush, I would not have written this book if it were not for you. I am achieving what I only dreamed of because of your encouragement.

Debbie, you are my amazing editor who makes my writing sound so eloquent and makes me laugh.

Mom, Dad, and my siblings Kathy, Sonya, Jim, and Tim, thank you for putting up with my "spirited" attitude as a child and believing in me for all these years. The Christian love from home is in my heart always.

Jillian, you are "my partner in crime" who suggested, "Maybe you should look into life coaching," and put the bug in my ear.

Rafael, you are my friend who helps me understand the Bible and are always there for me.

My son and daughter, Nick and Megan, you are both amazing and I am truly blessed! I cannot believe you are young adults already! You have always supported me no matter what. The Bible stories we read together as you were growing up were only the start of the strong faith in God I have seen mature in both of you. There were numerous times when your faith gave

7

me strength when I was weak. I could not ask for anything more! I know you will read this book from cover to cover!

Efren, you are my husband and so much more. . . Your support is incredible. You have given me the courage to change, step out, find what God wants, and then just do it. You are always there for me and continually backing me. Your child-like faith in God is incredibly inspiring and contagious and your love for life is unspeakable.

And last, Sierra, you have taken me back to who I am. The world that the love of a horse can take you to is understandable only to those who have experienced it.

Table of Contents

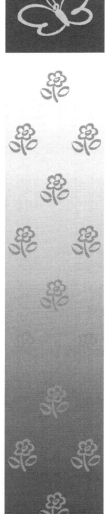

Free Gift For You!

Please go to
pammaldonado.com/free-gift
to download your
free gift!

To your amazing health and
happiness in body, mind and
spirit!
Pam Maldonado

Introduction

Psalm 139:13-16 (NIV)

"I praise you because I am fearfully and wonderfully made;

Your works are wonderful, I know that full well."

As someone who has spent a lifetime in awe and amazement of the human body, Psalm 139:14 has been dear to my heart and resonates with my soul.

The scripture is largely about the incredible nature of our physical bodies! The human body is the most complex organism in the world, and this complexity, amazing detail, and uniqueness shouts to us about the awesomeness of our Creator. Every detail down to the tiniest microscopic cell reveals that the body is indeed fearfully and wonderfully made!

Think about the human brain. It has the ability to learn, reason, control automatic functions of the body like heart rate, blood pressure, breathing, and balance at the same time we are concentrating on something else! When we put on glasses that turn things upside down to the eye, the brain automatically changes that information and gives us the perception that things are right side up. People who are blindfolded for a long period of time learn to use their vision center for other functions. For those who live next to the railroad tracks, the brain eventually filters out the noise and they lose conscious thought of it. The brain – fearfully and wonderfully made!

And think about this. The information needed for replicating the human body, every single detail, is all stored in the double-helix DNA strand found in the nucleus of each cell of the human body. There are billions of cells! With our ever improving microscopes showing us smaller and smaller fields, the unending discoveries of the human cell become more evident and more amazing. Imagine how much information is stored in something we cannot even see with our own eyes! The single cell – fearfully and wonderfully made!

The nervous system is a system of information and control. It is compact when we compare it to our manmade wires and optical boxes. Each simple cell of the body, so very tiny, is actually a small yet elaborate factory. The central nervous system – fearfully and wonderfully made!

Think about the single fertilized egg of a brand new baby forming in the mother's womb. From that one cell, forming in the womb of the mother develops all the various kinds of tissues, organs and system and they all work together at just the right time! The reproduction system – fearfully and wonderfully made!

What about the immune system? It has the ability to fight off diseases and restore itself from the tinniest cut to broken bones or injuries from major accidents! The healing capacity of our bodies – fearfully and wonderfully made!

How about the contrast of being able to handle large, heavy objects to the tiniest, most fragile thing without breaking it? Just think about how many things we do without consciously thinking about it? Keyboarding. Walking. Riding a bike. The musculoskeletal system – fearfully and wonderfully made!

The digestive tract, the respiratory system, major organs, nerves, blood vessels, the lymphatic system, cleansing of blood through kidneys, intricacies of the inner and middle ear, sight, smell, taste, feel...these are only the proverbial tip of the iceberg to all the amazing miracles of the human body. We truly are fearfully and wonderfully made!

You may not have paused to ponder the too-numerous-to-list spectacular functions of the human body until now. When you start to more deeply appreciate the miraculous body you have been given, it will be difficult to do anything less than your highest and best work toward wellness. Living with abundant health and wellness is the best way to glorify God through the miraculous body, mind and Spirit that He has given us!

Be blessed as you embark on this new journey. It is my prayer that your love and appreciation for the body your Creator has entrusted to you will translate into a ministry that helps you and the people you love live in complete abundance.

Pamela Maldonado, M.Ed., MCLC

Chapter 1: Overview of Wellness

Hear My Heart

I have been a physical education and health teacher for nearly 30 years. My appetite for new information leading to optimal health is insatiable. It is my passion to help others achieve and maintain wellness, and I am energized by the challenge of identifying the unique needs of each person committed to reaching those goals. As a Christian, I believe God expects us all to care for the bodies in which the Holy Spirit dwells. I love how the straight talk of *The Message* speaks to this expectation:

1 Corinthians 11:29-32 (NIV)

"For those who eat and drink without discerning the body of Christ eat and drink judgment on themselves. That is why many among you are weak and sick, and a number of you have fallen asleep. But if we were more discerning with regard to ourselves, we would not come under such judgment. Nevertheless, when we are judged in this way by the Lord, we are being disciplined so that we will not be finally condemned with the world."

It breaks my heart, and I believe God's as well, to see people created in His image living health-impoverished lives. And it saddens me to know that so much of this suffering is optional! I recently heard about a woman who was diagnosed with multiple sclerosis, and then three years later ran 366 marathons in 365 days. How

Wellness begins with personal responsibility and choices. What we choose to eat, drink, think, and believe largely determines the strength of our immune system and general health.

many of us would have used the same diagnosis as an excuse to retire from running? Consider the young men and women returning from Afghanistan with war injuries but determined to live life to the fullest regardless of their limitations. So many of these heroes adapt to their new challenges and embark on modified fitness training programs. In other words, nearly everyone, regardless of circumstances can be intentional about improving or maintaining health and wellness.

If you are reading this book, you likely share my enthusiasm for wellness coaching. Our desire is to help people reach their goals as they increasingly lean on God and His principles of abundant living. Unlike our secular counterparts, we are concerned with our clients' spiritual health in addition to their physical well-being. Though healthcare reform has been a topic of much debate in the United States, I think the following is an insurance policy we can all embrace:

Psalm 37:3-6 (MSG)

*"Get insurance with G*OD *and do a good deed, settle down and stick to your last. Keep company with G*OD*, get in on the best. Open up before G*OD*, keep nothing back; he'll do whatever needs to be done: He'll validate your life in the clear light of day and stamp you with approval at high noon."*

So, let us get to work, devouring all we can to help everyone created in God's image to be all He created them to be!

What is Christian Wellness?

There are so many definitions of wellness that if you researched them your head would spin! Therefore, using my knowledge, education, life experience, work experience, common sense, and most importantly, the influence of the Holy Spirit, I have created my own list of characteristics that I believe define Christian wellness. Before we take a look at those qualities, it is important to understand a foundational concept: wellness is personal and individual.

I encourage those I coach to approach wellness as if they were competing in an individual sport. Compete only with yourself, continually striving to set new personal best accomplishments. If you have ever gone on a diet with a friend at the same time, you know why this is so important. No two bodies are the same, and it is unrealistic, even demoralizing, to compare wellness goal attainment with other people.

Wellness begins with personal responsibility and choices. What we choose to eat, drink, think, and believe largely determines the strength of our immune system and general health.

Christian Wellness Is . . . .

- **A Choice:** *You* make the decision to move toward the best health possible for *you*.
- **A Way of Life:** *You* design this lifestyle to reach *your highest potential* for well-being.
- **A Process:** *You* develop awareness that wellness has no end point, is ever-changing with life, and is attainable in each moment.
- **A Combination of Body, Mind, and Spirit:** *You* acknowledge that everything you think, feel, believe, and

do creates a consequence – good or bad, for your state of health.

and finally. . .

· **Loving and Accepting Yourself as a Child of God:** *You understand and accept that you are fearfully and wonderfully made by God.*

Psalm 139:13-16 (MSG)

"Oh yes, you shaped me first inside, then out; you formed me in my mother's womb. I thank you, High God—you're breathtaking! Body and soul, I am marvelously made! I worship in adoration—what a creation! You know me inside and out, you know every bone in my body; You know exactly how I was made, bit by bit, how I was sculpted from nothing into something. Like an open book, you watched me grow from conception to birth; all the stages of my life were spread out before you, the days of my life all prepared before I'd even lived one day."

Components of Christian Wellness

Let us take a look at an overview of the components of Christian wellness found in the appendix of this book.

The goal of Wellness is to provide services that lead to a well whole person. The diagram is helpful for understanding how all areas of health and wellness are related. The components that are orange are the ones covered in the Wellness Coaching Course. You can see how everything is all tied together and that wellness is a matter of balance in all of these areas. And as you can see, it all comes from and feeds into God.

Spiritual Wellness: your ultimate meaning and purpose in life; congruity between values and behaviors which are based on Jesus Christ

Physical Wellness: your activities that help you keep your body in top shape and performance level which impact specific areas of your physical health such as weight control, exercise, nutrition, and sleep.

Mind/Intellectual Wellness: activities that encourage you to explore the world around you, learn more about yourself, and expand your mind in any way such as reading, learning new skills, taking part in hobbies, being creative, and sharing those skills with others

Emotional/Social Wellness: your emotional strength that forges your inner workings that foster healthy relationships and give you tools to solve and handle stress; how you see yourself in the world and in society; how well you adjust to changing roles; how well you deal with others and feel about yourself;

how you contribute to the environment and community; how you improve the world by participating in healthier lifestyles

Vocational Wellness: how you feel about your work; maintaining a positive attitude toward your job; enjoying a rewarding and enriching career path

Financial Wellness: how you manage whatever resources you have; your financial stability.

Medical Wellness: action you take to promote good health; regular medical checkups; preventative care

Who Needs Wellness Coaching?

According to the Center for Disease Control (CDC):

- Chronic disease is linked to 7 out of 10 deaths in America each year.
- Heart disease, cancer, and stroke account for more than 50% of all deaths each year.
- Chronic disease accounts for 75% of the $2.8 trillion in annual health care costs.

Now, a chronic disease is a disease that persists for a long period of time – generally about three months or more according to the U.S. National Center for Health Statistics. Chronic diseases are usually non-communicable illnesses that do not resolve spontaneously, and are rarely cured. Examples of chronic diseases include heart disease, cancer, stroke, diabetes, and arthritis. They are among the most common, costly, and preventable of all health problems in the United States. But, one thing we know for sure is that health damaging behaviors - particularly tobacco use, lack of physical activity, and poor eating habits - are major contributors to the leading chronic diseases. (Staff, 2012) This fact reminds us once again that wellness is largely a choice.

More than ever before, humankind -- the crown of God's creation -- needs Christian wellness coaches. God is summoning us to lead His people out of self destruction to become healthy, vibrant, and able to carry out His mission in their lives.

How many people do you know who want to quit smoking? Exercise more regularly? Eat healthier foods? Relax more? Spend more time with God? The desire to change is at the heart of coaching. Every one of those people is a potential client, and they represent a large percentage of the adult population in this country.

More than ever before, humankind – the crown of God's creation – needs Christian wellness coaches. God is summoning us to lead His people out of self destruction to become healthy, vibrant, and able to carry out His mission in their lives. Your job is to ask God to guide you as you do educate yourself through this course, and allow the Holy Spirit to guide you through the task He is equipping you to handle. I truly believe this is a Spirit led profession, and God is training you to lead those who need you.

And *ahhhhh*, the satisfaction you will feel when you hear. . .

> **Matthew 25:21** (NIV)
>
> *"His master replied, 'Well done, good and faithful servant! You have been faithful with a few things; I will put you in charge of many things. Come and share your master's happiness!'"*

The Correlation between Wellness, Health and the Bible

In order to be an effective Christian wellness coach, one has to understand what wellness is and its correlation to Christian principles. The Word of God has much to say about health and wellness. Throughout this book you will become familiar with many biblical references to help you in your coaching. These are great verses, and there are many more that are helpful for your clients. Most people do not think of going to the Bible for this advice.

Many clients find a Biblical basis for decision-making influences their commitment to change. When the connection is made that what they are attempting to do is possible because it is in accordance with God's will for them to live abundantly and full of health, energy, and vitality all with the purpose of glorifying God.

Scriptures Referencing Body and Mind

Romans 12:1-2 (NIV)

"Therefore, I urge you, brothers and sisters, in view of God's mercy, to offer your bodies as a living sacrifice, holy and pleasing to God—this is your true and proper worship. Do not conform to the pattern of this world, but be transformed by the renewing of your mind. Then you will be able to test and approve what God's will is—his good, pleasing and perfect will."

Coaching Application

Our bodies are so important that we are to offer them as a living, sacrifice, holy and pleasing to God. Think about that statement. Do you treat your body as a living sacrifice, keeping it in its best condition, nurturing it with proper rest, exercise, nutrition and love? Are you supplying it with everything it needs to be holy and pleasing?

I like to think that the way we tend to a newborn baby is a good way to think about how we should treat our bodies. Just think about it for a minute. You want to give that new life the best chance at life that is possible. You are responsible for the life of that child. You are the one taking care of this little temple of God, and as a result make sure he or she gets proper rest, food, love, snuggling, cuddles, baths, safety, and cover that child in prayer. You would not feed a baby fast food no matter how hungry they were. You would find the time to obtain the proper nutrition instead. Why do we do less for ourselves?

God has commanded us to take care of our bodies. Period. And, He commands us to take care of them in a way that is holy and pleasing to Him. Take some time to think about this mandate and how you take care of your body. This could be life changing!

Paul spoke passionately about the body being the residing place for the Holy Spirit:

1 Corinthians 6:19- 20 (NIV)

"Do you not know that your body is a temple of the Holy Spirit, who is in you, whom you have received from God? You are not your own; you were bought at a price. Therefore honor God with your body."

More from the Word . . .

On Weight Control

Proverbs 23:20-21 (NIV)

"Do not join those who drink too much wine or gorge themselves on meat, for drunkards and gluttons become poor, and drowsiness clothes them in rags."

I Corinthians 10:31 (NIV)

"So, whether you eat or drink, or whatever you do, do all for the glory of God."

On Exercise

Proverbs 31:17 (NIV)

"She sets about her work vigorously; her arms are strong for her tasks."

Proverbs 24:5 (NIV)

"The wise prevail through great power, and those who have knowledge muster their strength."

On Nutrition

I Timothy 4:3-5 (NIV)

"They forbid people to marry and order them to abstain from certain foods, which God created to be received with thanksgiving by those who believe and who know the truth. For everything God created is good, and nothing is to be rejected if it is received with thanksgiving, because it is consecrated by the word of God and prayer."

On Stress

Philippians 4:6-8 (NIV)

"Do not be anxious about anything, but in every situation, by prayer and petition, with thanksgiving, present your requests to God. And the peace of God, which transcends all understanding, will guard your hearts and your minds in Christ Jesus.

Finally, brothers and sisters, whatever is true, whatever is noble, whatever is right, whatever is pure, whatever is lovely, whatever is admirable—if anything is excellent or praiseworthy—think about such things."

On Sleep and Rest

Psalm 127:2 (NIV)

"In vain you rise early and stay up late, toiling for food to eat, for He grants sleep to those He loves."

Matthew 11:28 (NIV)

"Come to me, all you who are weary and burdened, and I will give you rest."

On Relationships

Hebrews 10:24-25 (NIV)

"And let us consider how we may spur one another on toward love and good deeds, not giving up meeting together, as some are in the habit of doing, but encouraging one another—and all the more as you see the Day approaching."

Your Purpose, His Plan

My prayer is that you will find peace and contentment in your next steps and be able to move forward boldly knowing that this is what God has called you to do. If He wants you to do it, there is no one who can stop you!

Sometimes it takes a while to know what God wants. And sometimes we find out what He wants by trying things that do not work out so well for us. I believe showing us what He does not want is as important as finding out what He does want. He is constantly honing me into the person who is willing to follow His next command, His next assignment, and His next mission – all to glorify Him. I am becoming stronger, bolder, more willing, and more convicted with each step I take.

But it still is not easy – at least not for me. He has pointed out to me innumerable times how my lack of patience and stubborn will to just do it myself needs to be tamed. God and I have a great relationship. I think He has a good laugh when I admit, ""Okay. So, I tried it my way and, yes, once again you have shown me that Your way is better. But could you have just told me that in the first place?" I know His reply is, "I did, but you didn't listen!"

I have learned that God will help you, but you have to start moving in order for Him to guide you. If you just sit there and wait for a message to be written on the wall or listen for a loud voice to shout your marching orders, like me, you too will miss it.

My brother once told me: God will only give you as much as you are ready for and sometimes it is like walking in the pitch black, dark night with a tiny flashlight, the kind that is on your keychain so you can see the lock on your car door. With this tiny light pointing down at the ground, you can only see what that circle of light allows you to see. If you go too fast, you will trip and fall and if you stop moving, well, you go nowhere. God only allows you to go as fast as He wants you to go and to see what He wants you to see.

Like pieces of a puzzle, He will give a piece or two at a time and it is up to you to put the pieces together. Think about how cool it would be at the end of our lives to look back and see it all as a completed puzzle? The final picture contains your whole life. Would all the puzzle pieces be there or would there be pieces missing? Those are the pieces we refused to use or were too busy, hurried, angry, lonely, hurt, haughty or obstinate to use. It's time we find all the pieces and put them to use. God has called us to help one another. This is your time to find out how!

As a Christian Wellness Coach, your purpose is to help your client seek individual wellness as it is aligned with God's purpose for them. In order to do this, you have to do this yourself! After that, you will be able to confidently help your client. Seeking God's purpose as you walk hand in hand with God and your client is a humbling calling.

In the Wellness Coaching Course, (www.pccca.org/ wellness) you will receive the information needed to complete the "Talk with God" activity which will be a major part of your Personal Wellness Coaching plan at the end of the Wellness Coaching Course. When you are finished, you will have a plan put together by you and God, created just for you!

The result will be amazing!

Chapter 2: Weight Loss

Oh how we have come to abhor this topic! Most people have dealt with this at least once in their lifetime and many of us are thinking about those extra pounds we should be losing as I write this sentence!

One thing I have learned is if you can insert a bit of humor into the quest for weight control, it becomes a bit easier to forgive yourself when you do not follow your plan. Humor also helps us realize that we are not perfect nor do we live in perfect bodies! And speaking of perfect bodies. . .remember the "perfect-body pictures" we see all over the Internet, on magazine covers, and plastered onto billboards are edited to remove cellulite, dimples, hills, valleys, wrinkles, and pimples. Ah, if it were only that easy in real life.

Admit it. Perfection is unattainable. So let us focus on what is realistic. If we embrace the key concept introduced in chapter one, we can begin to implement a lifestyle that begins with personal responsibility and choices. I think one of the problems we have is in the way we approach our attempts to control weight. We embark on a "weight loss plan" or "follow a diet." What you "lose" you will always be looking to find, and a diet reeks of deprivation and rigidity. Who wants that?

Before we get too far into the topic of weight loss, let us indulge in a bit of humor. I just love this little poem and it is best if you read it out loud. Everyone in your household will think you are fervently praying for weight loss.

The Dieter's Prayer

Author Unknown

Lord, my soul is ripped with riot, incited by my wicked diet.
"We are what we eat," said a wise old man. Lord, if that's true,
I am a garbage can.
To rise on judgment day, it is plain, with my present weight, I
will need a crane.
So grant me strength that I may not fall, into the clutches of
cholesterol.
May my flesh with carrot-curls be dated, that my soul may be
polyunsaturated.
And show me the light that I may bear witness,
to the President's Council on Physical Fitness.
And at oleomargarine I will never mutter, for the road to hell
is paved with butter
And cream is cursed; and cake is awful; and Satan is hiding in
every waffle.
Mephistopheles lurks in pepperoni, The Devil himself in each
slice of bologna.
Beelzebub is a chocolate drop, and Lucifer is a lollipop.
Give me this day my daily slice, cut it thin and toast it twice.
I beg upon my dimpled knees, deliver me from Jujubes.
And when my days of trial are done, and my war with malted
milk balls won,
Let me stand with Heavenly throng, in a shining robe – size 30
long.
I can do it Lord, if you'll show to me, the virtues of lettuce and
celery.

Teach me the evil of mayonnaise, and of pasta a la Milanese.
And crisp-fried chicken from the South, Lord, if you love me,
shut my mouth!

Now, at the risk of giving you emotional whiplash let me say something extremely important: I know there are many people for whom this topic is not very funny. I know the pain experienced by those people who have tried virtually every weight-reduction technique known to mankind without experiencing lasting results. Then, adding insult to injury is that natural process none of us can avoid called aging!

There are so many factors that influence our weight and an unending array of programs that claim to work. We are not created alike. We are all different. We have all arrived at this stage of our lives through different circumstances. So, will one program work for all? No, but we have to start somewhere with our clients. This wellness program assumes most people are typical, and we will ultimately coach to the exceptions.

For example, as a matter of routine I have all clients record what they consumed along with what they did for physical activity. It provides a great baseline for what we will do next. It is not uncommon to learn that despite eating a healthy, clean, nutrient-rich diet with reasonable portions and regular exercise, some clients do not realize the expected success. We then have to conclude that either the client was not being completely truthful with us, or there must be another issue to consider. This is the point at which you and your clients start working to determine what is causing the weight issue, and then explore options to overcome the challenge.

Here is a perfect example: I coached a client who wanted to lose weight. As we progressed through our sessions we found an underlying issue that as we soon found out, was actually causing the weight gain and therefore standing in the way of her achieving her goals. Her problem was that she would never voice her opinion in fear that she would cause a problem. This happened in her professional life as well as her role as parent and wife.

You are the only person who can affect change in your life. You are responsible for what you do, think, say, and believe. Without your commitment, there will be no change.

When she did not voice her opinion, she became angry. As a result, a huge undertow was created in her life and was one of the foundations she used to build all kinds of negative talk about herself and her own image. Once we started dealing with this issue and totally dropped the weight loss thing, she started losing weight. In fact, she lost 12 pounds in two months doing absolutely nothing different towards a diet or exercise plan! So, as you will find out more in the wellness course (www.pccca.org/wellness), we will be discussing a variety of options and avenues to use in order to help your clients become successful in living a life of abundant health and wellness.

In order to understand how to lose weight, we first have to understand why we cannot. Turn to the appendix and take a look at figure two, which is a reflection of some of my brainstorming. First of all, we start with the problem, which is the inability to lose weight. As you see on figure two, below "weight loss" there are three typical reasons people have problems losing or controlling their weight.

1. Eating Too Much,
2. Moving Too Little
3. Choosing Calorie-Loaded Foods

Yes, there are others, but for the majority of people, the problem usually falls within these three categories. So, let us examine why we default to these bad habits.

Why We Eat too Much

Emotional Eating

We may eat when we are nervous, anxious, frustrated, angry, lonely, feeling sorry for ourselves, and so forth.

Focused on Food

We may be focusing on food all day long. The more we try not to think about food, the more we tend to think about it, right?

Lack of Preparation and Planning

If we do not have a menu for our meals or have the food prepared or on hand, then when we just start foraging for whatever is in sight. By the time we make a meal, we have already grazed ourselves through an entire day's worth of calories.

Why We Move too Little

Rationalization

So often we have excuses as to why we do not move more. "I am in a hurry." "I just do not have the time." "This illness I have keeps from moving." "Why should I? There are a lot of people who do not and look how happy they are." And so forth..... I am sure you have come up with your own reasons why you just do not exercise or take the stairs instead of the elevator.

Automation

Advancements in technology have really taken a toll on the human body. Designed to make life easier and more productive, it has done just that. We can get most of what we want while sitting in a chair. I remember when I was a kid and we had to get up to change the channel on the TV and we also had handles in the car where you actually roll down the windows by hand! The phone had a cord on it and most of us only had one in the entire house, so every time the phone rang, someone had to get up and go to the phone to answer it. Just think of all the things we do not physically have to do anymore. The automated advancements are wonderful, but we now must be more deliberate about moving our bodies to keep it healthy. God created the human body to move and when it does not move, eventually it will not move!

Why We Choose Calorie-Laden Foods

Lack of Knowledge

First of all, many people are totally unaware that the supposedly "healthy" granola bar is full of sugar disguised in words so long they cannot be pronounced by the human lips! Nor do they know that most white flour is processed in your body like it is sugar and thus deposited as fat on the belly and thighs. Or that many of the ingredients in the conveniently packaged foods are foreign to the body and the body doesn't know what to do with it. We assume if it is on the shelf of the grocery store it is food. Evidently the definition of "food" has changed! You will get more on this later. How are you to know that when the package says "natural" that doesn't mean all the ingredients in it are "natural" and what does "natural" really mean?

Lack of Discipline

It is just much easier to grab a packaged meal or go through the drive-through for dinner – especially when you are in a hurry. But too many of us are in a hurry all the time so this becomes a daily lifestyle for us rather than a once in awhile treat. Once a person realizes what is being eaten in these convenient foods, the discipline may get a bit better. Sadly, for some of us, this discipline will become a matter of life and death!

Assumptions about Cost

Most people feel it costs too much money to eat healthy foods. I mean, the deals they have at the fast food places, many restaurants, and supermarkets are amazing – especially for those who have large families. However, the depressing part is, if you do not pay for the food your body can use for optimal health now, you will pay for it later in life in medical bills!

As you progress in your wellness coaching experiences, you will find this simple chart is a great tool to help clients begin to understand and identify their eating habits. Ask them questions like:

- Where do you fit into this table?
- Which characteristics fit your eating and moving lifestyle?
- What modifications could you make that would have the biggest impact on your overall wellness?

Then put on your investigator hat to determine "why" certain behaviors occur.

- Who is involved with you?
- How are you feeling at the time?
- What is happening at the time?
- When is this occurring?
- Where is this occurring?

- Who is influencing you to make these choices?
- Who are you with when you do this?

Simply a Decision

Controlling or not controlling our weight is simply a decision. And, it is a decision every person has made whether they acknowledge it or not. Making a decision to not exercise is a decision to not get stronger physically. Making a decision to eat junk food is a decision to eat more calories than is needed most likely gain weight. The only relevant question is whether or not your decision is leading you to the outcomes you want to see.

If you think about it, most things we do in life begin with a decision. Once you really make the decision to do something it is as good as done. So it is with weight control. The decision is half the battle and once the mind is made up, the mind prepares the body to obey. But is it so easy? Read carefully, and really listen to what Paul has to say:

Romans 7:14-25 (MSG)

"I can anticipate the response that is coming: "I know that all God's commands are spiritual, but I am not. Isn't this also your experience?" Yes. I am full of myself—after all, I've spent a long time in sin's prison. What I do not understand about

myself is that I decide one way, but then I act another, doing things I absolutely despise. So if I cannot be trusted to figure out what is best for me and then do it, it becomes obvious that God's command is necessary.

But I need something more! For if I know the law but still cannot keep it, and if the power of sin within me keeps sabotaging my best intentions, I obviously need help! I realize that I do not have what it takes. I can will it, but I cannot do it. I decide to do good, but I do not really do it; I decide not to do bad, but then I do it anyway. My decisions, such as they are, do not result in actions. Something has gone wrong deep within me and gets the better of me every time.

It happens so regularly that it is predictable. The moment I decide to do good, sin is there to trip me up. I truly delight in God's commands, but it is pretty obvious that not all of me joins in that delight. Parts of me covertly rebel, and just when I least expect it, they take charge.

I've tried everything and nothing helps. I am at the end of my rope. Is there no one who can do anything for me? Isn't that the real question?

42

The answer, thank God, is that Jesus Christ can and does. He acted to set things right in this life of contradictions where I want to serve God with all my heart and mind, but am pulled by the influence of sin to do something totally different."

I love this scripture because it says it like it is! To really get the full effect, go back through this scripture thinking about a specific problem and read it as if you are writing these statements about yourself. It is amazing how it works for every aspect of our lives. Here's an example for you:

Personalized **Romans 7:14-25** (MSG)

"I can anticipate the response that is coming: "I know that all God's commands are spiritual, but I am not. Isn't this also your experience?" Yes. I am full of myself—after all, I've spent a long time in sin's prison __eating late at night when I really do not feel good after doing that__. What I do not understand about myself is that I decide not to __eat at night any more__, but then I go and do it anyway, doing the thing I absolutely despise. So if I cannot be trusted to figure out what is best for myself and then do it, it becomes obvious that God's command is necessary.

But I need something more! For if I know I shouldn't **be eating late at night**, *but still cannot do it, and if the power of sin within me keeps sabotaging my best intentions, I obviously need help! I realize that I do not have what it takes. I can will it, but I cannot do it. I decide to* **stop eating late at night**, *I do not really do it; I decide not* **to eat like that anymore**, *but then I do it anyway. My decisions, such as they are, do not result in actions. Something has gone wrong deep within me and gets the better of me every time.*

I mess up so regularly that it is predictable. The moment I decide to do good, sin is there to trip me up. I truly delight in God's commands, but it is pretty obvious that not all of me joins in that delight. Parts of me covertly rebel, Like **my mind craving some food** *and just when I least expect it, they take charge.*

I've tried everything **to stop eating like that** *and nothing helps. I am at the end of my rope. Is there no one who can do anything for me? Isn't that the real question?*

The answer, thank God, is that Jesus Christ can and does. He acted to set things right in this life of contradictions where I want to serve God with all my heart and mind, but am pulled by the influence of sin to do something totally different."

Do you see how this can apply to anything? When you use this type of Biblical application with your clients, they also get the feeling that the Bible really does hold the answers to so many of our problems if we only search and find them, God is willing to be there and help us through our problems. The Word literally becomes active and alive in them! We must transfer this relationship with food into a deeper relationship with God. Take a few moments to think about the following:

· How does the amount of time and energy you spend thinking about food compare with the time and energy you spend thinking about God?

· What would our life be like if we spent as much time on God as we did on food?

· What might happen if all you did was follow these four simple steps?

  1. Eat *only* when you are physically hungry

  2. Eat *only* until you are full

  3. Eat *only* food that gives life, meaning food that is alive and nutritious

4. Drink half your weight in ounces of water daily

God has given us knowledge to know when and how much to eat. But we have conditioned ourselves to override this knowledge and follow our own desires, ultimately paying the consequences of poor health. If we follow God's laws, we will have abundant health.

Overeating also affects our friends and family. When we live our cavalier lifestyle in front of them, they also begin to think that these choices are okay. What would our lives, *and the lives of those we love,* look like if we spent this time with God instead?

How is it that we have squandered away what on the surface seems so simple to achieve? I believe we have lost control and feed our selfish desires so much that the "desires" God has placed in us are choked out, forced into the recesses of our brains never to surface again. Can we get that back? In reality, it is so easy to eat what your body needs. It is all about listening to your body. But I think we have forgotten (if we ever knew in the first place) how to listen. Here is something you can do to help you listen to your body, because, trust me. It is talking to you when you eat a certain food; think about how you feel after eating it. Do you have any of these symptoms?

Irritability
Hungry
Nauseous
Heavy
Sleepy
Lethargic
Energized
Just Right
Happy
Depressed
Headache
Stomach
Ache
Loose stools

Constipation
Rash
Achy Joints
Restless
Strong
Perfect
Jittery
Panicky
Paranoid
Coughing
Sneezing
Throat Crud
Itchy Eyes
Watery Eyes

We must transfer
this relationship
with food into a
deeper
relationship with
God.

I think you get the picture. You are listening to your body and how you feel will tell you how beneficial that food was for you. If you feel anything negative, then that food was not good for you. Food should make you feel good and equip you to do God's work. It should not make you want to take a nap, spend your afternoon running to the bathroom, or taking antacids. If your meal is speaking to you for minutes or hours after consumption, that particular food was not what God intended for your particular body to be eat for optimal health and wellness?

That being said, it is time for a little true confession. I *love* my husband's homemade beans; just *love them*! I know that every time I eat them, I will be miserable for the rest of the day. They will affect my intestinal tract for the next 48 hours, meaning I will be feeling like a blimp the whole time, grumpily going about my activities.

It is not only stupid to sacrifice 48 hours of productivity, crabbiness, and irritability for a taste that lasts for only a few minutes. It is selfish. I lose my best performance for God for the next 48 hours, and I also affect the wellness of those I work and live with!

But yet, as Paul talked about in Corinthians, we do the very thing we do not want to do and we know that we are doing it, but we do it anyway, just for a few minutes of ridiculous pleasure! We cannot control anything but by the power of the Holy Spirit, because that will to do the opposite, the sinful side of us, overtakes our good intentions.

We need to call in our only hope, Jesus Christ and His teachings. We must lean on them heavily, follow His advice, and win this battle. We must look outside of our sinful selves and look to God.

Accountable to God

We are personally responsible to care for our earthly bodies – the temple of His Holy Spirit. He is a jealous God, who commanded us to love Him with all our hearts, and soul, and strength. When we put any other passion ahead of Him, we are being disobedient. God wants us to worship Him and Him alone.

Given all the false idols available to us, we fall short of His will. Money, food, sex, sports, drugs, TV, Facebook, stuff, status, and so many other things have become our passions, and ultimately our gods. God has asked us to live a life completely devoted to Him, the ONE AND ONLY GOD! You can choose to worship the Creator or what He created. Jesus' words, "not my will, but yours be done" (Luke 22:42 NIV) have been forgotten and neglected by so many Christians.

Taking personal responsibility for your own behavior will lead you down the narrow road, but it will be the major freeway that will make all the difference in your life and your life's mission for God! How you control your weight and live your life is your choice: day by day, meal by meal, step by step, thought by thought.

Is it easy? Not at all. And if anyone tells you it is, they must have been one of those lucky people who never had much of a weight control problem, and God bless them for that!

Keep it Simple!

I have found that people who want to start eating better are more successful once they have the mindset, discipline, right reasons, and motivation for reaching a healthy weight. Simplify all of these factors, making it more realistic to attain goals.

Focus on lifestyle change – not diets, calories, protein, fat grams or diet foods. Only eat what your body is asking for – regardless of what you are tempted by in your environment. Stop eating to reward yourself or just feel more comfortable. Focus on God and His plan for you more than your focus on food. Listen to your body to eat the amount of food that is right for you. By the power of the Holy Spirit, be personally responsible to God as a caretaker for your body, exercising the fruit of the

Spirit (love, joy, peace, patience, kindness, goodness, faithfulness, and self-control).

When I saw Jesus on the movie *The Bible*, I was struck by how little Jesus thought about eating! His main concern was doing His Father's work! Think about that in contrast to our habits. I, for one, would love to be more like Jesus in this regard, and I know we can.

One of the activities in this course is "My Secret Affair: Is This a Healthy Relationship?" exercise about eating. This activity will be "huge" in your quest to get "small." (Did you catch that little joke there?)

You are the only person who can affect change in your life. You are responsible for what you do, think, say, and believe. Without your commitment, there will be no change. Once again, this is easier said than done, but it is 100% doable when you lean on God! Here are some tips to help you do just that.

Visualize your perfect, God-given self. Take a few moments to jot down some key words that will help keep this vision in front of you. Make sure the things you desire are the same things God desires for you. Shift your focus from food, to God's will for you. The sooner you do this, the sooner you will lose weight. Change your thinking about food. Eat to live instead of living to eat.

I thought it might be interesting for you to see what a friend of mine does to control her weight. This is just an example of one person I know who tries to keep her weight control very simple and something she can easily call her "lifestyle."

- Eats **s**lowly
- Makes healthy choices
- Cooks from scratch
- Eats processed foods in moderation
- Exercises regularly
- Moves a lot during the day
- Doesn't obsess over food
- Eats something sweet when she wants to
- Enjoys her food
- Always works to get more physically fit – not just stay thin

She has clearly found what works for her. What would be on your list? Would my friend's way of thinking about weight control be any different from yours? Ask your clients the same question. The behaviors we ultimately demonstrate are first created in the mind. Help your clients see how their thinking may be sabotaging their success. In fact, this is such a powerful tool we will spend much more time on the topic later in this book. For now, let us try to harness some of the power and rewrite our life's script.

Created Twice

Everything in this world is created twice; first in the mind, and then physically. An architect creates blueprints and plans before the house is actually built. A car is created on the engineering desk before it hits the assembly line. You are created twice, also.

Yes, God planned and created you. But that is not what I am talking about here. I am talking about the way we have created ourselves – first in the mind, and ultimately in reality. For most of us, there is quite a mismatch from God's intention to our persona.

As a young child, you were created as those people whom you interacted with infused you with beliefs, beliefs about yourself and your surroundings. They may have told you that you were no good, that you were trouble, would never amount to anything, or worthless. You may have been abused, told the world was ugly no matter where you went, that you were too fat, ugly, and no one would ever want you. Sometimes the messages are more subtle. How many overweight girls heard, "You have such a pretty face, if only...." and you know how the sentence is finished.

Some people carry those scripts with them throughout life. But now, as an adult, and particularly as someone who knows the love of God, you have the chance to rewrite your script. If you have already done this work, congratulations for stepping out of the label bondage. If you have not, take some time to think about those tapes that play in your head that you are unconsciously living out. Here is a little exercise to get you started.

1. Think new thoughts.
2. Clarify new thoughts with words.
3. Put new words into action
4. Make your actions become habits.
5. Let your habits define your character.
6. Watch your character lead you to your destiny.
7. Realize your destiny with more abundant life in Christ.

Here is a practical example of this concept: Linda was the oldest of six children. She was the chubby one, always compared to her younger, smaller-framed, and thinner sisters. In fourth grade her doctor put her on diet pills. It was the 60s, and everyone was taking them then. They worked for a while, but like every diet, the weight always came back on, plus a little more. Her entire lifetime was spent trying every diet under the sun. Eventually she decided to just give up. After all, she was the chubby one and some things just do not change.

Now that Linda knows this is an unhealthy script, she knows she can create a healthier one. She has a **thought** and asks herself, "Is my health really only defined by the number on the scale or the size tag in my pants?" She attaches **words** to her thought. "I can be healthy even if I am overweight." She translates her words to **action**. "I could walk for 20 minutes a day." She commits to make her action a **habit**. "I will walk 20 minutes a day for five consecutive days a week." She begins to see that her new habit is forming her **character**, "I am a disciplined woman who is increasing credibility through commitment." She recognizes that her newfound character is leading her to her **destiny**. "I am healthier today than when I started walking, and in the process, I've even lost a little weight."

Linda's destiny has led to a more abundant life in Jesus Christ. "I truly can do all things through Christ who gives me strength. And now I have a body that has the stamina it needs to do all God intended for me to do for His glory."

There you go. A simple example of what I said earlier, that everything is always created twice, first in the mind and then in reality.

Set the Stage for Results

Resist the urge to skip the step of engaging your brain in the change process. I will bet you have tried that before and it didn't work well, or you would not be reading this book. This is not to say you need a perfect plan before you begin, but you do need something you can visualize doing. Come up with something you like, appreciate, or in this case with weight loss, what you want to look like. Maybe a picture from years ago of yourself, or a picture from a magazine or computer that has the type of physique you want as your "blueprint" so to speak. It is something for which you can aim – a vision in your brain to keep you moving in the right direction.

Please remember this tip: in order to change, you must write out your plan – not type it on the computer, you can do that later – but you have to actually write it down so that your entire body acknowledges the thought and understands it. This simple act will propel you to your new life!

In the webinar for this chapter, I show students a diagram that helps them envision change, especially as it pertains to lifestyle choices. It makes all of what I have been talking about quite simple and easy to start implementing into you or your client's lifestyle.

Affirmations – Your Go-To Panic Button

Positive affirmations are first-person, present tense statements about how you want to feel, look, think or act. They have been scientifically proven to help people reach their goals, dreams, and desires. Affirmations combined with Biblical truths are extremely effective in influencing human behavior.

How does this work? We all have heard thousands of negative statements in our lives. These statements paralyze our inner belief and keep us from reaching our potential. At some point, these statements are "affirmed" enough that our subconscious mind believes them. This is the point in our lives that we begin to own our unique negative self-talk.

"I am so _____ (fill in the blank) stupid, fat, irresponsible, fearful, angry, sad, incompetent, and so forth

These are short, powerful statements written in the present tense –statements of fact. "I fear nothing, because perfect love casts out all fear." "I am positive and optimistic because God does not test me beyond my ability to endure." "I am loved because I am fearfully and wonderfully made."

Try writing a couple. Decide what you want to do, find scripture to complement your goal, and write affirmations to support it.

The death and life of your success and your dream is in the power of your tongue. If you keep speaking the same words, you will keep getting the same results. Affirmations help you to speak life! To change your life, you must change your words. Start by making a conscious decision to speak to the solution instead of the problem. Memorize Bible verses of victory. Start with these.

Proverbs 8:21 (NIV)

"Death and life are in the power of the tongue..."

Matthew 12:34b (NIV)

For the mouth speaks what the heart is full of.

Proverbs 6:2 (NIV)

You have been trapped by what you said, ensnared by the words of your mouth."

Mountains can be moved with your words! Do not just speak to God about how big your problem is. Speak to your problem about how big your God is!

Mark 11:22-23 (MSG)

"Jesus was matter-of-fact: "Embrace this God-life. Really embrace it, and nothing will be too much for you. This mountain, for instance: Just say, 'Go jump

in the lake'—no shuffling or shilly-shallying—and it is as good as done. That's why I urge you to pray for absolutely everything, ranging from small to large. Include everything as you embrace this God-life, and you'll get God's everything. And when you assume the posture of prayer, remember that it is not all asking. If you have anything against someone, forgive—only then will your heavenly Father be inclined to also wipe your slate clean of sins. "God is bigger than any obstacle you face! Oh, what power we have been given through Christ! We just have to speak it and get rid of what the world has been telling us. Do not conform to the world!"

So, you know that God wants abundant health and life for us. Therefore it is okay and you can give yourself permission to say it and believe it! That can be an affirmation for you if you want.

You can take a negative thought...I am so fat! And change it into a positive affirmation that says..."I am lean, beautiful, strong and full of energy and vitality"! As you say this out loud, over and over again, you will begin to erase the "negative way" that you are thinking about yourself, which in essence, is how you are actually telling yourself you will be! If you say, I am fat, then, you are fat! And so you will stay that way because you are giving your body, mind and soul no other alternative! But, if you say "I am lean, beautiful, strong and full of energy and vitality!" Guess what...you are and you will be!!!! You are AFFIRMING who you want to be!

Keep these statements that affirm who you are in your phone, index cards or any place where you can have them with you for the situation when you just want something so bad and you know you will feel awful if you give in to it!

You could have this list on the fridge at home or on your mirror in the bathroom to see every day when you get up or stuck on the dashboard or visor of your car...just have them all over the place so you can constantly be reminded of the proper way to think for success!

If you look, there are unending sources of affirmations you can get off the Internet and in books, or better yet, just write your own! The only rules are that they must be positive and they must be written in the first person. Here are five affirmations I really like.

1. My body is getting leaner, stronger, and healthier every day.

2. My body deserves love and kindness, and so I treat it that way.

3. I believe I can lose weight and keep it off.

4. I enjoy eating nutritious food and taking care of my body.

5. I am worthy of healthy food and deserving of a healthy body.

More Techniques for Desperate Times

Following are a few more techniques to use when you are tempted to eat something unhealthy or to give up:

Breathe and count. Slowly count to 10 and then take 10 deep breaths. Now decide whether or not you are still going to make an unhealthy choice. Many times, by the time you get to your fifth breath, the urge has passed and you feel so good that you made the right choice.

Remind yourself of why you want to get or stay healthy with a picture. This picture may remind your clients that not only do they want to take care of themselves for themselves, but also so they can be a spouse, parent, friends, or co-worker.

Find motivational quotes and hang them where they will be seen. I like these two from Isabel de los Rios:

"Every choice you make either gets you closer to your goal or further away from your goal.
Which way do you want to go today?"

or

"When you feel like quitting, think about why you started!"

In the webinar training (www.pccca.org/wellness) we will participate in an exercise to creating positive affirmations and changing your negative thoughts into positive affirmations that will change your thinking! Also, you will be able to get all of these "extras" as downloads to be able to use for yourself or to compile for your personal use as a Christian wellness coach.

Chapter 3: Exercise

It is estimated that Jesus walked about 21,595 miles in His lifetime. The distance around the equator is 24,901.55 miles! Wow!

What is the purpose of exercise?

God created the human body to move. When we do not move, we lose the ability to do so. Quality of life is greatly enhanced through exercise. Consider just a few of the benefits of moving. Moving lightens your heart, gives you time to walk and talk with God, increases bone strength, relieves stress, burns fat, builds muscle, and increases stamina for daily activities. That extra dose of strength becomes increasingly important as we age, and exercise will help with coordination, balance, and flexibility.

*It troubles me that only three out of 10 people actually take or should I say **make** time to do this. [exercise] I would be willing to bet, that most of those people are very successful in other areas of their lives as well. Successful people know the value of discipline and the value of health.*

And think about the sense of accomplishment you feel when you have followed through with exercise, even though you may not have wanted to do it.

So, how much bang for your workout buck do you really get? Well, there are many studies out there, but we are going to look at one recent study in particular. Then you can make your own decision about the importance of exercise if you really want to keep God's temple in tip-top shape. One of the primary questions people ask about exercise is, "If I exercise, will I live longer, and if so, how much longer?" This study addresses that question.

Brigham and Women's Hospital and the National Cancer Institute have attempted to answer this question by quantifying how much longer people live depending on the levels of exercise in which they engage. After following about 650,000 subjects for an average of 10 years and analyzing more than 82,000 deaths, they were able to draw the following conclusions.

The researchers found that people over 40 who participated in different levels of physical activity and with varying amounts of body mass benefited with a longer life span. To sum it up, generally speaking, the more you exercise, the longer you will live.

For example, 75 minutes of brisk walking per week equates to an extra 1.8 years of life expectancy for as opposed to those who remain more sedentary. Increase that to 150–299 minutes of brisk walking per week and the gain in life expectancy goes up to 3.4 years. Make it 450 minutes per week and the estimated life expectancy jumps by 4.5 years.

The study also found that people whose weight is above the recommended level still benefit from physical activity. Men, women, normal weight, and overweight people all benefit from exercise in terms of longevity. However, the best results were obtained by exercisers of normal weight. People with a normal body mass index (BMI) of 18.5-24.9 added 7.2 years to their life expectancy when compared with people with a BMI of 35 or more with no exercise.

There are numerous studies that have arrived at the same conclusion. One study claims you gain seven minutes of life for every minute you exercise, and if you increase the intensity of the exercise, the effects are magnified. It has also been proven that people who exercise live longer, healthier, and far more productive lives than those who are sedentary.

As we age, we become more interested in these kinds of statistics. We realize how weak we can get and how sad life can be if we choose to undermine our bodies and shorten the time fulfilling God's plan for our lives. But it is never too late to do *something!* Another study I read reported on a 70-year-old man who did strength exercises combined with a cardio workout and gained as much muscle mass as a 40 year old! This result was verified by comparative MRIs. So, you see, there is hope for you and your clients. It does not matter how old you are. Now is the best time to implement an exercise program because you will benefit from it!

What are the benefits?

- Healthier Heart
- Higher Levels of High-Density Lipoproteins (HDL, the good cholesterol)
- Increased Lung Capacity
- Decreased Risk of Many Cancers (including breast and colon cancer)
- Improved Job Performance and Fewer Sick Days
- Stronger Bones
- Clearer Skin
- More Energy
- Better Sleep
- Easier Menstrual Cycles
- Decreased Anxiety, Stress, and Depression
- Weight Loss, Decreased Appetite, More Efficient Metabolism
- Stronger Ability to Fight off Illnesses Such as Diabetes

- Slower Aging Process
- Improved Mental Ability
- Digestion and Elimination
- Prevents Cold and Flu
- Decreased Pain and Improved Arthritis
- Quicker Recovery from Illnesses Injuries, and Surgeries
- A More Positive Outlook during Recovery
- Improved Confidence and a Feeling of Independence
- Studies suggest that people who start exercising in their sixties can significantly reduce the risk of developing Alzheimer's in their seventies; the risk drops even further if they start exercising in their forties or fifties.

Despite all these positives, only three in 10 American adults get the recommended amount of physical activity, according to the <u>President's Council on Physical Fitness and Sports</u>. The best way to exercise is to do something that keeps you active every day! But remember. Get the okay from your doctor before starting any exercise program to make sure you are healthy enough to do this!

How Much Should You Exercise?

This is a general outline of a very basic program you can build upon. It is a good place to start if you or your clients have not been doing much physical activity. Walking is always a good starting place and easy to do as it requires no equipment or special clothing.

The CDC says adults should get at least 150 minutes a week of moderate-intensity aerobic activity such as brisk walking. There are a lot of ways to look at a goal such as this:

· It could be 30 minutes a day, five days a week
· It could be 75 minutes a week of vigorous activity such as jogging
· It could be a mix of both moderate and vigorous intensity aerobic activity each week.

In addition to what is stated above, add two days each week of strength training activities. You will realize more benefits for having done so.

If you have not been active for awhile, start out slowly by walking 10 minutes two times a day and then increase to 15 minutes two times a day. Soon you will be up to 30 minutes a day, five days a week to meet the

In my opinion, every exercise program should incorporate moving every day in some way that will cause you to huff, puff, and sweat. And, moving your body in a variety of ways that mimic daily movements for living is a benefit as well.

minimum guidelines. If you then add the two days of strength training, you will be meeting the minimal guidelines set by the CDC. In the appendix of this book, you will find a chart provided by the CDC that you can use with your clients. This is a good place to start for anyone who is just beginning an exercise program.

That example of exercising just gives you a guideline of where to start. It is only a minimum! Everyone is different and has a different reason to exercise. It troubles me that only three out of 10 people actually take or should I say *make* time to do this. I would be willing to bet, that most of those people are very successful in other areas of their lives as well. Successful people know the value of discipline and the value of health.

It is also interesting to think about the same statistic this way. Though 30% of Americans are exercising regularly, 70% of us are not. That means 70 % are thinking short term, and that never works for the long term. There are consequences to this decision.

You have heard the statement "pay me now, or pay me later." The short term mentality says survive now and do not think about the future. The long-term thinkers know that if they pay now with just 30 minutes a day, five days a week, they will not only live longer, but will be productive basically all those years!

Short-term thinkers can look forward to less appealing outcomes.

So what kind of exercise is right for you and what is out there?

Think about yourself first; what is important to you and what do you want to achieve out of this? For example, in my case, I am very busy and a bit hard-core about exercise! I grew up on a dairy farm and knew what hard work was, but I also understood how much more fun it was to play if I was strong, fast and nimble. I got a lot of that running for my life from my older brother! And yes, I deserved every bit of what he gave me, however, I found that I was far ahead of my classmates in physical fitness and that was because my lifestyle on the farm was constant motion!

Far different than my "townie" friends who had no idea how fast they could run if a mad cow was chasing you! I mean, if you think about what you did as a kid, jumping, running, climbing, crawling, pulling, throwing, walking, I mean really, what if we did now what we did then?

Well, in essence, that is what a lot of workout programs mimic. But you see, as a child, it was play and as an adult, it seems to be work, why? You can answer that one, but in order to follow an exercise program that is consistent and lasts a lifetime, you have to think of it as fun! You must create it or have someone help you create a "fun" way to work out or chances are you will not do it.

My personal idea of exercise is that I need to sweat and huff and puff as hard as I can or it is not even worth it! Once I have done that, then I will go for a walk or something more relaxing to me. However, my life has been athletics, exercise, games and working out! As a college athlete of two sports, all I did was work out and study! I had to in order to be good enough to play at the level that I wanted to play. That is just me. To me, that was fun!

You and your clients may be very different from me. I have some clients that when they started, could not walk more than 10 minutes, and there was no way they could get down onto the floor let alone get back up again. So you see we need to have some good experience in all kinds of exercise in order to help people of all different abilities, desires, and physical capabilities.

In my opinion, every exercise program should incorporate moving every day in some way that will cause you to huff, puff, and sweat. And, moving your body in a variety of ways that mimic daily movements for living is a benefit as well. Everyone needs to start with functional exercise, and then make it a goal to go above and beyond.

What do I mean by functional? It is completing the day-to-day tasks of daily living: walking, standing up, sitting down in a chair, picking things up off the floor, getting down onto the floor and getting up, putting things up on a shelf, carrying groceries, getting in and out of the car, pulling, pushing, lifting, twisting, turning, bending, and so forth. Just think of all the ways you move in a day and how you want to be able to maintain that activity until the day you die. An optimal exercise program will keep you functional and fit, well into your golden years!

Many of the workouts I recommend and practice incorporate functional movements with free weight, body weight, stability equipment and cardio all wrapped up into one intense, 12-15 minute full-body workout.

What that means is for the 12 -15 minutes of the workout, the workout is as intense as is comfortable for you. This time is divided up into short "bursts" of hard work and rest. It burns energy that is stored in the muscle during the workout and burns fat to replace that energy after the workout and your heart and lungs get an amazing workout as well. You will build core strength, flexibility, coordination, and balance. Each workout is different over the course of the weeks and months so the body does not adapt.

The best part about these exercise programs is that anyone can do them regardless of age or physical ability. You chose the movements that you are capable of doing and increase their difficulty as the body gets stronger. You may not be able to do a push up, but a good coach can show you how to adapt them so you can start out with wall push-ups, then progress to hands on the couch, then to push-ups slightly elevated, until you can do a regular one. Every exercise can be adapted to work for your particular ability.

Maybe you cannot do squats which are wonderful exercises for developing the large muscles in your lower body. You can start sitting in a chair and practice standing up and sitting down using whatever you need for assistance to accomplish that. While one person may be doing squats with weights on their shoulder, I may be doing regular squats. You can do them along with me doing your own form of squats, using a chair, or against a wall with a stability ball. There are so many ways to exercise in order to fit your own personal ability!

So, for burning fat and toning up the body, check out this research to help support short, intense workouts. Researchers at Laval University in Quebec divided the participants into two groups: long-duration and interval, short-term exercisers. They had the long-duration group cycle up to 45 minutes without interruption. The interval, short-term group cycled in numerous short bursts of 15–90 seconds, while resting in between. The long duration group burned twice as many calories, so you would assume they would burn more fat.

However, when the researchers recorded their body composition measurements, the interval group showed that they lost the most fat! In fact, the interval group lost nine times more fat than the endurance group for every calorie burned!

Here is another example.

Control Trial: The Twin Study

Dr. Al Sears conducted a study on female twins.

Kristen did progressively more long endurance exercise in each session, while Lauren did progressively shorter bursts of intense exercise, increasing the intensity in each session, too. In the sixteen-week course of the study, the twin doing interval training (short bursts)lost 13 pounds of fat and increased her muscle mass by eight pounds. Her body fat fell from 24.5% to 14.2%. The twin doing long bouts of aerobic exercise lost only seven pounds of fat and gained only one pound of muscle mass. Her body fat fell from 24.5% to 19.5%. Neither of these women became bulky, but the twin doing interval training had a much better tone to her look at the end of the study. You can find the study at this website.

Here is how it would look in a treadmill, elliptical, outdoor walking, running or actually any type of movement that you would want to do. You could do jumping jacks, burpees, rope jumping, or walking steps if you wanted to. It is up to your imagination! You may be surprised!

It is my passion to help everyone exercise to accomplish wonderful health and maintain it until we die. At least that is what most of us want -- to die young as old as we can!

If you are using cardio equipment like an elliptical or bike, you do not need to reach any "magical" speed. It is highly individual, based on your current level of fitness. But you know you are doing it right when you're exerting yourself to the point of typically gasping for breath, after a short burst of activity.

An added boon is that you will save a tremendous amount of time because this type of workout will cut your hour-long cardio workout down to a total of 20 minutes or so, including your recovery time, warm-up, and cool down.

The actual sprinting totals only four minutes! Here is what a typical routine might look like using a recumbent bike, treadmill, walking, or sprinting outside. Warm up for three minutes. Exercise as hard and fast as you can for 30 seconds. You should feel like you could not possibly go on another few seconds. Recover for 90 seconds. Repeat the high intensity exercise and recovery seven more times. Be mindful of your current fitness level and do not overdo it when you first start out. If you are not in great shape and just starting this you may want to start with just two or three repetitions, and work your way up to eight, which is where the magic really starts to happen. You may need to start with just walking and when you do your 30 second bursts your legs would be moving as fast as possible without running, and your arms would be pumping hard and fast.

If you can do this type of work out twice a week, and follow a healthy eating plan, you will increase your production of growth hormone, and this burns fat. Once you regularly participate in these 20 minute exercises about twice a week, most people notice the following benefits:

·   Lowers your body fat
·   Dramatically improves muscle tone
·   Firms your skin and reduces wrinkles
·   Boosts your energy and sexual desire
·   Improves athletic speed and performance
·   Allows you to achieve your fitness goals much faster

There are four additional types of exercise that will turn your workout regimen into a truly comprehensive exercise plan:

1. **Aerobic**: Jogging, using an elliptical machine, and walking fast are all examples of aerobic exercise which will increase the amount of oxygen in your blood and increase endorphins, which act as natural painkillers. Aerobic exercise also activates your immune system, helps your heart pump blood more efficiently, and increases your stamina over time.

2. **Strength Training**: Rounding out your exercise program with a one-set strength training routine will ensure that you are really optimizing the possible health benefits of a regular exercise program. You need enough repetitions to exhaust your muscles. The weight should be heavy enough that this can be done in fewer than 12 repetitions, yet light enough to do a minimum of four repetitions. It is also important not to exercise the same muscle groups every day. They need at least two days of rest to recover, repair and rebuild.

3. **Core Exercises:** Your body has 29 core muscles located mostly in your back, abdomen, and pelvis. This group of muscles provides the foundation for movement throughout your entire body, and strengthening them can help protect and support your back, make your spine and body less prone to injury, and help you gain greater balance and stability. Pilates and yoga are great for strengthening your core muscles, as are specific exercises

you can learn from a personal trainer, though a personal trainer may be out of reach for you right now.

4. **Stretching**: My favorite types of stretches are active isolated stretching (AIS) http://www.stretchingusa.com/ developed by Aaron Mattes. It is an amazing way to get flexibility back into your system, and it is completely different from the traditional type of stretching.

No one should have the excuse that they cannot. They can. However, it may be in a different way than what is considered traditional, and God has given us a brain and a will to determine what that may be in order to help so many struggling individuals who really want to be well and fit!

It is my passion to help everyone exercise to accomplish wonderful health and maintain it until we die. At least that is what most of us want – to die young as old as we can! Think about that one!

We can all be lifting weights in some form whether in the form of exercise bands, body weight, free weights, weight machines, cans of soup, an eight-pound gallon of water, or a sack of potatoes. It is life and we need to live it to our best as we are living within the guidelines that God gave us this body, His temple, and it needs to work hard – in fact it *likes* to work hard!

Can you over exercise? Yes and many people do. You must listen to your body. Pain and muscle soreness that does not go away is a sign of over exercising that many people ignore. If you are feeling exhausted, do not exercise as hard or just take a rest day. The benefits of exercise are cumulative. It is what you do over a lifetime that matters, and the time is now!

Also do not let your life be run by exercise. Again, as I have said in the other chapters, a healthy balance is what wellness is all about. Obsessing about exercise puts everything out of balance. God must be your number one God. Do not replace Him with exercise! I have been guilty of doing so in the past. I used to run my day by my workouts. It was nuts and not good for the soul!

Incorporating Working Out into Your Day

Find five-minute increments to exercise every single day. Studies show that 20-30 minutes of exercise is all that is needed to see significant health benefits and changes in your body. The best news is that time can be split up over the day as needed. For example, if you get in four, five-minute workouts in one day, that is just as beneficial as getting in one 20-minute workout. Great news, right? But do not lose sight of nutrition!

You cannot out exercise a poor eating plan! Period!

Exercise does not always balance out eating too much food or the wrong kinds of food. Exercise may not always work for your weight loss plans

The best part about these exercise programs is that anyone can do them regardless of age or physical ability. You chose the movements that you are capable of doing and increase their difficulty as the body gets stronger.

Also, this is very important...because you have a genetic disposition to disease doesn't mean you have to have that disease as exercise and good nutrition will combat that most of the time!

Guidelines for Setting up an Exercise Program for Wellness

The main goal is for your clients to move. Period! To what capacity they move, is where you begin. Make a list of goals, reasons they want to start or change their exercise program. You must ask a lot of questions to help them to come up with the reasons why, how, and to what intensity this program should be done. If they come up with the idea themselves as a result of your questioning they are three times more likely to follow through! An exercise program must be fun, motivational, and challenging. In the end, such a program will lead them to a lifetime of abundant health and achievement of their pre-ordained purposes so that they can keep doing the work that God has asked them to do and not grow weary!

As a coach, you must:

- Hold them accountable
- Give them motivation
- Enthusiasm
- Praise
- Encourage them to share what they do with others.

As we all know, if you teach what you know, it will become even more engrained into your being. So if they branch out to help someone else, they will be held even more accountable and will enjoy even more success as they will start to actually live what they are practicing thus the chance of embedding a lifelong healthy habit to support that temple God has given us!

How to Set Up a Workout/Exercise Plan

When starting an exercise plan, there is a process to go through so that you or your client is assured of success!

Always make sure you or your clients are cleared by a doctor. Make sure you or your clients are healthy enough to begin an exercise program, especially if this person is someone who has not been working out before this or who is sedentary and suddenly beginning to work out.

In the Wellness Coaching Course (www.pccca.org/ wellness), I will show you exactly how to set up an exercise program for any client. You will be receiving a detailed list of what to include as well as forms and templates to use that will make this part of your coaching a breeze yet very, very effective for your client. This will be a great tool to help yourself or your client reach an optimal level of wellness. You will need that good health to do the work that you were sent to accomplish!

Chapter 4: Nutrition for Your Life

Blessing for Food

I love Dr. Don Colbert. He has written so many excellent books about health. It is not often you find material written by a medical doctor who quotes scripture and encourages adherence to God's laws within his works. Here is an excerpt from his book, *The Seven Pillars of Health, the "Natural Way to Better Health for Life.*

> *"Thank you for my wonderful food and its healing properties. Mark 16:18 tells me that if I drink [or eat] any deadly thing it shall not harm me. Thank You for protecting me supernaturally from any harm that may be in my food. I ask that You bless the food to my body according to Exodus 23:25, which tells me that "He shall bless my food and my water and He will take sickness away from the midst of me."*

> *I eat this food with thanksgiving. I receive His love and rejoice in the Lord as I eat my meal. As I eat this food, my cells, tissues, and organs are cleansed, strengthened,*

and renewed like the eagle. I see myself
healed. In Jesus' name, amen."

As we progress through this chapter, remember your responsibility to honor God by caring properly for your earthly body. Pay attention to your reactions to what you read. Use the following material to coach yourself to better wellness as you prepare to do the same for others.

Balanced Nutrition

Wellness is all about balance, and balance also applies to nutritional needs. Eating a balanced diet means choosing a variety of colors, textures, and types of food. Too much or too little of any food over an extended period of time throws our entire being off balance.

Let us say that you have two pantries in which to store your food. One pantry is labeled "Foods of Death" and the other is labeled "Foods of Life."

One reads:

"SIDE EFFECTS: May lead to chronic, degenerative diseases like arthritis, diabetes and heart disease. Typical reactions include weight gain, fatigue, susceptible to hypertension and high cholesterol which could lead to heart attack."

The other says:

"**SIDE EFFECTS:** May guard and protect against developing cancer, heart disease, most degenerative/chronic diseases and obesity. Typical reactions include increased energy, vitality, and a more youthful appearance."

One leads to death. The other leads to life. Which pantry appeals to you more? Nutrition and wellness are all about choice. It is interesting to see what average Americans are choosing to eat in a year. In an article entitled _Food Consumption in America,_ you can read some of the staggering statistics concerning the diets people choose. Figure V in the appendix of this book is a graph that summarizes the information detailed in the article.

The graph is a tool to use as a good starting point for coaching someone to wellness. Ask them which pantry they think most Americans go to when they are hungry. Discuss the foods specifically and make determinations about which pantry the foods should go into. Ask them what is in their pantry at home right now. This conversation will help you establish a nutrition knowledge baseline for your client. Plus, you will have an opportunity to introduce invisible potential threats like pesticides, growth hormones, and additives. There are few things in life where the choices are so simple: death or life. That is it. Every morsel of food either contributes to death or life.

The best description of death and life foods can be found in Dr. Don Colbert's book, *The Seven Pillars of Health, the "Natural Way to Better Health for Life.* Dr. Colbert makes the point that not all things we consume deserve of the "food" label. He urges us to choose living foods – those in raw, or close to a raw state such as fruits, vegetables, grains, seeds, and nuts. Living food even *looks* alive. God created our food with vitamins, minerals, phytonutrients, antioxidants, fiber, and more – all known to contribute to healthy digestive systems, bloodstream, and organs.

On the other hand, dead foods have been altered to stay on the shelf as long as possible and even cause addictions in people. Processing results in loss of nutrients and conversion from originally healthy foods to something man-made and even toxic to our bodies. Human tampering results in foods including preservatives, food additives, bleaching agents, and so on. Strain on the liver, stored fats, and plaque in the arteries are some of the many adverse effects on our bodies.

I hope you are beginning to understand why living food is so important to life. The majority of our illnesses are brought on by poor food choices. The pharmaceutical companies do not need to make an obesity vaccine or another magic pill. Start by choosing real foods of life.

What the Bible Says About Nutrition

Eating a balanced diet in moderation is supported in nearly every nutritional plan you look at. However, the best book in the world, *The Bible*, gave us this nutritional plan, many, many years ago. When God fed the nation of Israel during its exodus from Egypt, he said:

Exodus 16:16-18 (NIV)

"This is what the LORD has commanded: 'Everyone is to gather as much as they need. Take an omer for each person you have in your tent.'"

The Israelites did as they were told; some gathered much, some little. And when they measured it by the omer, the one who gathered much did not have too much, and the one who gathered little did not have too little. Everyone had gathered just as much as they needed."

God told them to take enough to just meet their needs. This same principle is used again in the New Testament teachings of Jesus Christ in the book of Matthew where Jesus told them not to worry about what to eat as God would meet their needs.

Matthew 6:25-34 (NIV)

"Therefore I tell you, do not worry about your life, what you will eat or drink; or about your body, what you will wear. Is not life more than food, and the body more than clothes? 26 Look at the birds of the air; they do not sow or reap or store away in barns, and yet your heavenly Father feeds them. Are you not much more valuable than they? 27 Can any one of you by worrying add a single hour to your life?

Living between the extremes of starvation and gluttony is wonderful advice for your nutritional health!

10 Steps to Better Health

1. Stop drinking pop, especially diet pop!

Pop has no benefit to the health of your body. Check out what some leading doctors have to say about it in this article from *Off the Grid News* (July 2013). The real cancer risk from soda is sugar, which prominent physicians, including CNN's Dr. Sanjay Gupta and Dr. Robert Lustig of the University of California at San Francisco's Medical Center, call toxic. Another health expert, Dr. Joseph Mercola, noted that a typical can of soda contains the equivalent of ten teaspoons of sugar in the form of high fructose corn syrup. Mercola pointed out that colas contain so much sugar their manufacturers have to add phosphate to them to keep people who drink them from vomiting.

Check out the ingredients in soda. It is like reading a foreign language. By reading the ingredients, a person still doesn't understand what is in the pop, but there is one ingredient on the list that I need to point out; high fructose corn syrup. Though high fructose corn syrup does come from corn, it is chemically processed and changed from its' natural state so when you put it into your body, it is a chemical known to overwhelm your liver as explained in the following paragraph by Dr. Mercola. Dr. Mercola wrote in *Sugar May Be Bad, but This Sweetener Called Fructose is Far More Deadly* (January 2010): "Your body metabolizes fructose in a much different way from glucose. The entire burden of metabolizing fructose falls on your liver. And fructose in any form – including high-fructose corn syrup (HFCS) and crystalline fructose – is the worst of the worst! Fructose, a cheap sweetener usually derived from corn, is used in thousands of food

The majority of our illnesses are brought on by poor food choices. The pharmaceutical companies do not need to make an obesity vaccine or another magic pill. Start by choosing real foods of life.

products and soft drinks. Excessive fructose consumption can cause metabolic damage and triggers the early stages of diabetes and heart disease, which is what the Davis study showed." It is not like sugar, which also carries adverse effects for your body, and it is not like honey! It should be avoided whenever possible.

And there is more. Contrary to popular beliefs, diet soda also impacts nutritional health. There are some studies that suggest diet pop could be more damaging to your body than regular pop according to *Diet Soda Health Risks: Study Says Artificial Sweeteners May Cause Weight Gain, Deadly Diseases* written by Dominique Mosbergen and published in *The Huffington Post* (July 2013).

And then there is this: "Honestly, I thought that diet soda would be marginally better compared to regular soda in terms of health," Swithers, a behavioral neuroscientist and professor of psychological sciences, told CNN. "But in reality it has a counterintuitive effect." The researchers found that just like with regular soda, the consumption of artificially sweetened beverages like diet soda is also associated with obesity, type II diabetes, metabolic syndrome and cardiovascular disease. Drinking just one can of diet soda per day is "enough to significantly increase the risk for health problems," according to the media release. Some of the health issues associated with soda consumption include obesity, diabetes, heart disease, liver damage, insomnia, high blood pressure, osteoporosis, and various cancers.

Sharon P. Fowler, MPH, and colleagues at the University of Texas Health Science Center, San Antonio, looked at eight years of data from 1,550 people aged 25 to 64. "What didn't surprise us was that total soft drink use was linked to overweight and obesity," Fowler reported. "What was surprising was when we looked at people only drinking diet soft drinks, their risk of obesity was even higher. There was a 41 percent increase in risk of being overweight for every can or bottle of diet soft drink a person consumes each day."

Artificial sweeteners in diet soda can trick you into thinking you are getting something sweet for free, but your brain is not fooled. Most sweet foods have calories. Sugar substitutes do not have calories. By providing that sweet boost to your brain, but denying the calories, your body actually craves the calories you are denying it, leading to snacking, overeating, and obesity.

There is so much to cover on this topic and during the Wellness Coaching Course, (www.pccca.org/wellness) we will learn how this "sweet yet deceitful" product can affect so many aspects of a person's health and overall well-being and can potentially and profoundly change the life of your client! It is actually amazing!

2. Whole Fruit...YES! Just Juice...NO!

While fruits and vegetables are incredibly healthy, if you take just the juice out of them, you leave behind things like vitamins, minerals, fiber, and antioxidants. God created most of these foods to be eaten whole, and He created these foods to work together in our bodies to create good health. When we eat just part of the food, we are predisposed to imbalance. Store purchased juices are usually loaded with sugar that will add to the likelihood of contracting any of the many illnesses associated with over consumption of sugar. These illnesses are listed in the following article by Dr. Mercola. *"It is a poison by itself,"* Dr. Lustig says.

Dr. Mercola wrote in <u>Eliminate this ONE Ingredient and Watch Your Health Soar</u>, *"If Lustig is right, then our excessive consumption of sugar is the primary reason that the numbers of obese and diabetic Americans have skyrocketed in the past 30 years,"* the NYT says. *"But his argument implies more than that. If Lustig is right, it would mean that sugar is also the likely dietary cause of several other chronic ailments widely considered to be diseases of Western lifestyles — heart disease, hypertension and many common cancers among them."*

3. Sugar...NO!

"Sugar has been proven to destroy life and impair health. Over consumption of this poison has been linked to low energy, mood swings, hot flashes, restless sleep, migraines, anxiety, depression, mental fogginess, feeling out of control, inflamed gum disease, cavities in the teeth, aches and pains in the joints. These are really just the symptoms that people will typically feel when they consume too much sugar. These are all red flags that

Eating a balanced diet means choosing a variety of colors, textures, and types of food. Too much or too little of any food over an extended period of time throws our entire being off balance.

your body is trying to tell you something is wrong. When these red flags get ignored they can turn into full blown health conditions like heart disease, cancer, diabetes, arthritis and osteoporosis."

(Sources: The Health Detriments of Sugar Revealed, Dr. Peter Osborne, Gluten Free Society
Wed, 30 Nov 2011, http://www.sott.net/article/242236-The-Health-Detriments-of-Sugar-Revealed)

This is such an important subject to me I need to elaborate more on the dangers of sugar. I have read that for every American who eats five pounds of sugar each year, another person eats 295 pounds of sugar. I do not know where that statistic was generated, but I see it a lot. However, what I do know for certain is this: "Our ancestors ate about 22 teaspoons of sugar per year. The average American eats 150 to 180 pounds of sugar per year." (Mark Hyman: The dangers of sugar in all its forms, Greenmedtv.com, Wed, 06 Mar 2013) That is a believable statistic given that 69.2% of adults age 20 and over are overweight: (2009-2010)
http://www.cdc.gov/nchs/fastats/overwt.htm.

"I have seen clients and loved ones suffer from severe complications of type II diabetes. Over consumption of sugar and refined carbohydrates is a leading cause of type II diabetes. Processed sugar, which is in cakes, cookies, processed cereals, and many other foods, can literally be considered a poison, which is anything that directly causes harm and can lead to a diseased state when you ingest it." (Isabel de los Rios, Certified nutritionist, exercise specialist, bestselling author http://weightplanplc.blogspot.com/, July 22, 2012)

She also says that daily sugar consumption creates an acidic state in the body. The body's reaction is to fight this by pulling out minerals from bones, teeth, and other body tissues to fix this imbalance. This reaction relates to things like osteoporosis, tooth decay, and more. If the intake of processed sugar is not controlled, it will eventually affect every organ of the body. When the liver has stored all the sugar it can, the extra sugar is returned to the blood as a fatty acid. These fatty acids are stored as fat in the parts of your body that are the most inactive: belly, buttocks, breasts and thighs. When these spaces get filled up, it starts to deposit it in the heart, liver and kidneys which then lead to diabetes and diseases in these organs. Substitute things like stevia, raw honey, 100% maple syrup and xylitol whenever possible because these substitutes do not react in your body the same was as sugar does. Once again, we have just begun to scratch the surface. I recommend you do some of your own research on processed sugar. It may change your or your client's thinking.

4. Unrefined Sea Salt...YES!

You do not have to cut it out all together; just switch to a healthy form of it. Most salt research has been done on commercial table salt. Instead of this refined table salt, use unrefined sea salt or Himalayan rock salt. These are really healthy and have the exact opposite effects as refined table salt. They provide the perfect balance of minerals, nutrients, and sodium chloride that the body needs for optimum health.

5. Processed Food...NO!

Processed foods are really just science experiments and have no healthful food value whatsoever! Your body does not have a clue how to deal with them. Your liver is responsible for filtering your blood and it works like crazy to try to figure out what needs to be kept for the body to use and what needs to be filtered out. It gets overwhelmed trying to figure out these processed foods. It gets clogged and then it cannot process even "good" food effectively. This leads to weight gain.

(http://www.beyonddiet.com/Programs/BeyondDiet/Top-Ten-Mistakes/3-Lab-Experiments-should-not-be-considered-Food Isabel de los Rios)

If it is natural, meaning, if it grows or otherwise occurs in nature, eat it. If it is artificial, forget it! Do your liver a favor.

6. Bread...MAYBE!

Most bread is made of refined grains. White bread has had the essential vitamins and nutrients taken out of it during processing and wheat bread contains processed wheat, which is deficient in nutrients. These breads can be very inflammatory for many people. If you like to eat bread, try buying the sprouted grain breads. Or, if you want to make your own, get the unrefined flour or use the ancient grains like kamut and spelt.

Eating a balanced diet in moderation is supported in nearly every nutritional plan you look at. However, the best book in the world, The Bible, gave us this nutritional plan, many, years ago. God fed the nation of Israel during its exodus from Egypt.

7. Soy...NO!

Here are some facts about soy. Soy messes up a person's thyroid function, causes digestive problems, and attributes to mineral loss in bones. Soy also causes low energy, depression, hair loss, poor skin, weight gain, and lowered sex drive. I will bet you are surprised by this information, given the reputation soy has for being a healthy food.

8. Real Butter...YES!

Replace your artificial butter with raw, organic butter. This butter is actually one of the best whole foods you can include in your diet! Raw, organic butter helps maintain hormone balance, keeps arteries supple and flexible because of high lauric acid, encourages healthy glowing skin and hair, provides vitamins K, D and E, is rich in antioxidants, and more!

9. Canola Oil...NO!

This oil contains high amounts of erucic acid which is a fatty acid associated with heart disease. It is very unhealthy for your body. It is heavily processed, made from genetically modified seeds or also called genetically modified organisms (GMO) and when used in cooking with high heat, oxidizes and produces free radicals that can cause cancer and other diseases.

Instead, use unrefined coconut oil for very high heat cooking, and raw organic butter and olive oil for medium heat cooking.

10. Water...YES, YES, YES!

Our bodies are composed of about 75% water! Always drink half of your body weight in pounds in ounces daily. Example: 160 pound person should drink 80 ounces of water daily. Water regulates body temperature, flushes toxins, cushions joints, helps the body metabolize stored fat, and is a major player in helping the body get rid of waste, a natural laxative and a natural diuretic.

Foods to Eat for Life

- Organic Produce
- Raw Dairy in Small Portions or Substitute Coconut Milk
- Raw Nuts
- Whole, Preferably Sprouted Grains
- Water, Water, and More Water
- Healthy Oils Like Coconut and Olive
- Organic Butter
- Organic Protein
  - Fish (salmon, tuna, whole sardines)
  - Grass-fed Beef
  - Organic, Hormone-free Chicken
  - Whole, Organic Eggs

That is it. No prepackaged foods. No processed foods. Just good, naturally grown, hormone-free and pesticide-free foods that we were meant to consume in the first place.

Metabolism Types

One really important aspect to nutrition and wellness is metabolism. As a coach, you will want to become familiar of the different types. The three most common metabolisms are Protein Type, Carbohydrate Type, and Mixed Type.

Protein Type

People with a Protein Type metabolism have a stronger appetite than the other types. They enjoy fatty and salty foods and tend to think about food even when not hungry. They have a faster metabolism when it comes to oxidizing carbons. To regulate this process, they need higher amounts of protein as well as fats. Protein Types are often unsuccessful at skipping meals and fasting, which makes them irritated easily. Vegetarian and low-fat diets are not advisable for Protein Types unless you are very good about getting enough protein from those vegetable, nut and seed sources.

Carb Types

Carb Types tend to have weak appetites, are happy with minimal amount of food each day, and can get by on small amounts of food. They do not think about food much, eat less often, and may go for extended periods of time without eating. A Carb Type needs a diet composed of more carbohydrates than proteins or fats.

Mixed Types

A Mixed Type requires an equal balance of proteins, carbohydrates, and healthy fats, and including variety in the everyday meal plan is essential. Of the three metabolism types, this one is actually easiest to manage because the food choices are greater. Some meals may resemble those for Protein Types, and some may resemble those for Carb Types. Some meals may have features of both.

The appetite of a Mixed Type tends to vary greatly throughout the day—hungry at meals but not in between; extremely hungry at times and no appetite at others. This might help you to understand why you may have certain "cravings" or certain eating patterns that differ from friends and family members.

In the Wellness Coaching Course, (www.pccca.org/ wellness) I will be providing you with example meal plans for each metabolism type as well as resources for you and your clients to take a test and find out what your metabolism type is and a comprehensive list of foods that fit your specific type! You will be able to help a client come up with a "menu plan" that fits the liking of their taste buds as well as their metabolism type! Also, I will be showing you how you or your client's "eating plan" can work for the entire family. No more cooking separately! Just remember that no one plan works for everyone, and what is provided is just an example.

Organic Food

Organic food is grown or raised without the use of chemically formulated pesticides, herbicides, fungicides or fertilizers – allowed to grow in its natural state. In *How to Eat, Move and Be Healthy*, Chek (2004) lists the following chemicals found in a conventionally grown apple, a food that most of us would consider healthy!

- Chlorpyrifos: an endocrine disruptor that impairs immune response, causes reproductive abnormalities, and damages a developing nervous system
- Captan: a carcinogen (i.e., a substance believed to be capable of causing cancer) that causes genetic and immune system damage
- Iprodione: a carcinogen
- Vinclozolin: a carcinogen and a genetic, endocrine, and reproductive disruptor that causes dermatitis

Another study analyzed the urine of school children that ate a conventional diet and every one of them showed levels of pesticides in their urine that exceeded the Environmental Protection Agency's safe level.

When it comes to meat and eggs, what you eat can only be as good as what "it" ate. Cattle raised in lots are fed low quality grains to make them get fat faster. Since they are not designed to eat these grains, they get sick, so then they are given antibiotics. We ingest those same antibiotics when we eat grain-fed beef. Most chickens and pigs are raised in very small cages, usually in their own feces, and hardly ever see daylight. They too are fed a constant supply of antibiotics and hormones to speed growth and fight off diseases. This point alone should be enough to make you want to spend some extra money on free-range organic chicken and pork! I do!

Eggs will only be as good as the chicken that lays it. Chickens that live in a natural chicken environment produce eggs that have an extremely high level of omega-three fats which is one of the healthiest types of fat for people. The whole egg is one the healthiest, well-balanced natural foods for humans to consume. Many people are afraid of eating eggs because of the cholesterol in the yolk, but cholesterol is necessary for our bodies to function. The truth is eggs from commercially raised chickens are very high in omega-six fats which cause inflammation in the body and increase the risk of heart disease.

Is Organic Worth the Extra Cost?

I grew up on a farm. Our animals were never, ever in that type of environment. My father knew that healthy animals produced healthy food and there was no compromise in their food or conditions. Eating conventional food will eventually hurt your health. I would rather go with less than to subject myself and my health to eating food of poor quality. And, if I buy those products I am unintentionally supporting practices that result in unhealthy food.

You will save money when you stop buying processed foods, but even so, going organic can be a challenge for a tight budget. But it can be done. In the Wellness Coaching Course I will be supplying you with a comprehensive list of foods and showing you how to eat organically without the big price tag. This could be some of the most valuable information you can get from this course in order to help your clients achieve optimal health!

In the Wellness Coaching Course (www.pccca.org/ wellness), amongst other things, I will have available for you a daily food/exercise journal which is really nice for those who are serious about making changes in their nutrition plan. In order to really get a good handle on what you are eating, you have to write it down. Then, you can gradually start substituting the better choices into your plan. Do not forget, all of this pertains to your clients and the more you utilize this information yourself, the better you will be able to help your client. You will have the credibility of having "been there, done that" experience to share with them.

Chapter 5: Stress and Sleep

Emotional Health – Stress

Hold a glass of water and ask yourself, "how heavy is this glass of water?" Eight ounces? Ten ounces? Sixteen ounces?

The weight of the glass of water does not matter. What matters more is how long you hold it. If you hold it for about a minute, you should have no problems. If you hold it for one and a half hours, your arm will get achy. If you hold it for 30 hours, your arm will feel numb and dead. The longer you hold it, the heavier it becomes!

Stress and worry can affect us similarly. Hold on to stress for a short time, and not much will happen. Think about those stressors for a longer time, and you are going to experience discomfort. Obsess about them, and you will ultimately feel paralyzed, reducing your capacity to do much of anything. There is such a thing as good stress.

Stress is a natural reaction our body has to a perceived threat or dangerous situation. Stress is the gap between what you think is going to happen and what actually happens.

For example, a party you are putting on, a promotion,

birth of a child, or a wedding are examples of stressors that can actually be healthy. But we are going to focus on the stress that is not healthy. The longer you dwell on what is causing you stress, the more magnified it becomes and takes over your life. How you handle stress determines how much pain and heart ache you will experience. It is in your control, it is your choice!

Stress is a natural reaction our body has to a perceived threat or dangerous situation. Stress causes a quick release of adrenaline and other hormones that make your blood pressure rise, your heart start beating faster, and your lungs start pulling in more oxygen with more rapid breathing. There are several other physical changes that take place as well, but these are the ones we actually experience. These changes get you ready to fight for your life or to run for your life! You also get increased mental acuity, as well as all of your senses are heightened and you get extra strength to deal with the situation. This is great in a situation where you need it. Our caveman ancestors needed it to avoid saber-toothed tigers.

However, if this stress response happens too often or for a long period of time, those hormones that were supposed to save your life will start to work against you and cause harm. The very hormones that God created to save you in an emergency will actually start to kill you, slowly! Instead of helping you out of a jam, those stress hormones are causing you to feel depressed, anxious, and angry, have a low sex drive, and make you vulnerable to obesity, type II diabetes, high cholesterol, hypertension, and many other diseases!

The promise of this verse is just awesome!

Philippians 4:6-7 (NIV)

"Do not be anxious about anything, but in every situation, by prayer and petition, with thanksgiving, present your requests to God. And the peace of God, which transcends all understanding, will guard your hearts and your minds in Christ Jesus."

This verse pretty much tells us not to stress out about anything! Instead, be thankful and just talk to God about what you need and then "let go, let God." Paul writes that the peace of God we cannot understand will guard our hearts and minds. God has designed prayer as a stress reliever for your life problems. So, how do we let go? Before we answer that question, let us back up a bit and talk more in depth about stress.

What is Stress?

Stress is the gap between what you think is going to happen and what actually happens. Stress is how you deal with situations. It is response to changes, good or bad.

What Causes Stress?

Everyone has stressors in life. How you react to those stressors determines the level of stress you feel. Stress by itself is healthy until the weight of the stressors leads to distress. Busyness, lack of time, a family emergency, a new job, health issues, or any change, good or bad, can bring on stress. How you respond to these changes determines your stress level and your health. Following is a list of the various diseases caused by stress:

- Depression
- Headaches and Migraines
- Sleep Disturbances and Insomnia
- Backache
- Heart Problems
- High Blood Pressure
- Colds and Other Infectious Illnesses
- Stomach Ulcers
- Digestive disorders
- Chronic Fatigue Syndrome (CFS)

· Fertility Problems and Menstrual Cycle Disorders

Those were some of the problems stress causes. Now let us take a look at the signs or symptoms of stress. This information is a bit lengthy, but I felt it is important for you to be aware of as many signs of stress as possible for yourself and your clients.

Signs of Stress

Refer to the appendix for a list of common symptoms of stress. As I said earlier, some stress is good. Stress can cause us to get out of a dangerous situation or motivate us to get something done. Typically though, good stress is not chronic in nature, and usually has an end to it.

How does One Deal with Stress?

One of the simplest, yet hardest strategies available to us for dealing with stress is to change how we think about the stressor itself. Learn how to control how you react to the stressor. Learn how to calm yourself down and de-escalate the emotions.

Go to the Bible. Lean on God and remember to cast all of your cares on Him.

As a Christian wellness coach, the first place to start is with the Word of God. Meditate on them as He has given us the blueprint of how to live stress free.

Scriptures that help us deal with stress

Philippians 4:8 (NIV)

"Finally, brothers and sisters, whatever is true, whatever is noble, whatever is right, whatever is pure, whatever is lovely, whatever is admirable—if anything is excellent or praiseworthy—think about such things"

Mark 10:27 (NIV)

"Jesus looked at them and said, "With man this is impossible, but not with God; all things are possible with God."

Part of coping with stress is learning how to put it in the right perspective as this verse of "comfort" states so clearly.

2 Corinthians 1:3-4 (NIV)

"Praise be to the God and Father of our Lord Jesus Christ, the Father of compassion and the God of all comfort, [4] who comforts us in all our troubles, so

that we can comfort those in any trouble with the comfort we ourselves receive from God."

Colossians 3:15 (NIV)

"Let the peace of Christ rule in your hearts, since as members of one body you were called to peace. And be thankful."

God's plan is to bring peace to a troubled world at the return of Jesus Christ. We can have that peace now if we follow His plan for peace. It involves a lifestyle change and a change in our hearts. Peace is part of the fruit of God's Holy Spirit (Galatians 5:22) and finally,

I Corinthians 10:13 (NIV)

"No temptation has overtaken you except what is common to mankind. And God is faithful; he will not let you be tempted[b] beyond what you can bear. But when you are tempted, he will also provide a way out so that you can endure it."

Consider Biblical examples of people facing severe trials. Whatever the trial, when they asked God for help, He provided the strength and help for them to bear it. Jesus Christ Himself was "in agony" and "his sweat became like great drops of blood falling down to the ground" as He prayed before His crucifixion (Luke 22:44). God strengthened Him, and God will strengthen us as well when we ask.

Mindfulness is another way to diminish stress. Stay in the present. Experience life – moment-by-moment. Let go of thoughts unrelated to the moment. Find enjoyment in the here and now.

Matthew 6:34 (MSG)

"Give your entire attention to what God is doing right now, and do not get worked up about what may or may not happen tomorrow. God will help you deal with whatever hard things come up when the time comes."

Thankfulness and Gratitude are Examples of Mindfulness: A Psalm of David –Psalm 103:1-5 (NIV)

"Praise the LORD, my soul;
*   all my inmost being, praise his holy name.*
Praise the LORD, my soul,
*   and forget not all his benefits—*
who forgives all your sins
*   and heals all your diseases,*

who redeems your life from the pit

and crowns you with love and compassion,

who satisfies your desires with good things

so that your youth is renewed like the eagle's."

Reframing

One of the simplest, yet hardest strategies available to us for dealing with stress is to change how we think about the stressor itself. Learn to control how you react to the stressor.

Mindfulness is learning to stay in the present. Reframing is a way of changing the way you look at something and as a result, change your perception and experience. Reframing can change a stressful event into a major trauma, or it can make a stressful event nothing more than a new challenge to conquer. Reframing can change the attitude of a really bad day into just a mild low point in an overall beautiful life. Reframing is a deliberate decision to perceive a negative event as a learning experience. Reframing is a way we can alter our perceptions of stressors and, thus, relieve significant amounts of stress and create a more positive life before actually making any changes in our circumstances.

How Does Reframing Affect Stress?

Your body's physical response to stress is triggered by *perceived* stress – not actual events – and reframing will actually change your physical response to stress! Pretty cool! Reframing by using scriptures is one of the most powerful ways to deal with stress. Replace fear, worry, failure, grief, sorrow, and shame with God's promises!

Stressful thoughts damage the body and the Bible says that the mind is a "wellspring of life" and we need to change or reframe how we think about past events in our lives that we perceive as negative, ugly, painful, and so forth.

> **Proverbs 16:22** (NIV)
>
> *"Prudence is a fountain of life to the prudent, but folly brings punishment to fools."*
>
> **II Corinthians 10:5** (NIV)
>
> *"We demolish arguments and every pretension that sets itself up against the knowledge of God, and we take captive every thought to make it obedient to Christ."*

Romans 12:2 (NIV)

"Do not conform to the pattern of this world, but be transformed by the renewing of your mind. Then you will be able to test and approve what God's will is—his good, pleasing and perfect will."

Jesus said in the following...

John 16:33 (NIV)

"I have told you these things, so that in me you may have peace. In this world you will have trouble. But take heart! I have overcome the world."

Profiting from Trials

James 1:2-3 (NIV)

"Consider it pure joy, my brothers and sisters, whenever you face trials of many kinds, because you know that the testing of your faith produces perseverance."

Keep gratitude, peace, love and joy in your heart. The heart will control the brain and then the brain will control the thoughts. And the mouth will speak peace, gratitude, love and joy!

To sum up Dr. Don Colbert in *The 7 Pillars of Health*,

- Stay mindful of the present
- Be thankful to God
- Reframe everything that happens to you according to the truths of God's word
- Ask yourself, what did I learn from this experience to avoid it happening again?

Stress is basically in your mind and how you perceive the situation. If we keep our focus on God and know that He is in control, those stressful things will not seem as stressful and will only seem like a low point in a perfectly glorious day of that overall beautiful life we already mentioned. Again, wellness and how we perceive stress is a choice – our choice!

If you feel you want to have more detail or want to strengthen your coaching in the stress area, I suggest you go to http://www.pccca.org/stress.html for an excellent Christian Stress Relief Coaching opportunity where you can learn far more than we can cover in this time frame.

Sleep: Do you get enough Zs?

Consequences are always connected to our choices. Getting up early in the morning has little to do with setting the alarm or dragging yourself out of bed. What matters most is the time you went to bed the night before. Each decision affects another one. Levels of emotional stability, mental alertness, and physical endurance are affected by all of the choices we make. In this chapter we are going to become more aware of how our choices about sleep will affect our health and disrupt or improve our level of wellness.

In the 1800s people would get an average of 10 hours of sleep a night. In 1910 the number of sleep hours was down to nine, then eight in 1970 and less than seven in 1997. Most third world countries are still getting 10 hours of sleep. We, however, have changed that requirement mainly to become more productive at school and at work. Trying to juggle everything in life, work, family and leisure, we choose to take away from our rest and burn the candle at both ends.

Here are some fun facts about how many hours of sleep various critters need:

Koala Bear – 20-24	Horse and Elephant – 3
Cat – 16	Human, Rabbit, and Pig – 8
Dog – 15	Opossum – 19
Jaguar – 10	Mouse – 13
Chimpanzee – 9	Dolphin and Seal – 6
Cow, Sheep – 4	

How to figure out how much sleep you need? There are really only two things you have to do, but you will need to find the time to do it. Set a regular bedtime to stabilize your biological clock and create your environment so you are not "awakened" by anything in the morning. You want to wake naturally.

Write down when you wake up on your own each morning. If you have been sleep deprived you may sleep 10-12 hours or more the first couple of nights and then the amount of sleep you need will start to level off until you develop a regular number of hours each night.

I can already hear you saying, "When am I going to do that?!" I know that is hard for a lot of people, but it is really the only way to figure it out. I guess if you want to do it badly enough, you will find a way. Like all wellness-related issues, managing your sleep schedule is a choice!

Here is a story about a young man that burned the candle at both ends. Robert Murray McCheyne (1813– 1843) of Edinburgh, Scotland, was a young man ablaze with passion for Christ and His Kingdom. An ordained pastor of St. Peter's Church in Dundee when he was 23, McCheyne made such an impact that one listener said of him, "He preached with eternity stamped upon his brow. I trembled, and never felt God so near" (Rice, 2005). For the next six years McCheyne zealously and tirelessly presented the gospel of Jesus Christ to all who would listen. In 1839, he made a trip to the Holy Land to evangelize the Jews, and upon his return contributed to a great revival that swept across Scotland and northern England. Soon afterward, however, his health began to fail. Ignoring the urging of his concerned friends, he refused to rest and continued to push himself to the limit. Finally, as the young preacher lay on his deathbed at only 29 years of age, he whispered to a friend at his side, "God gave me a message to deliver and a horse to carry it. Alas, I killed the horse, and now I cannot deliver the message" (Sanders, 1997, p. 136).]

(Taken from Walters, Peter; Byl, John (2007-11-05). Christian Paths to Health and Wellness (Kindle Locations 7098-7101). Human Kinetics. Kindle Edition.)

That story is a great illustration to show that even if you are doing God's work you are not immune to the laws that He has put into motion. You cannot continually ignore rest for the body as this can be a fatal mistake! When God created the earth and all that is in and on it, He rested on the seventh day. Maybe we should be listening before we "kill our horse along with the message that we are supposed to deliver!"

We must understand our physical limitations. God has created and intertwined rhythms everywhere in His creation. There is the rise and setting of the sun and the moon, the tides, the different phases of the moon, the changing seasons as well as the circle of life with birth, growth, decay and death of all living things. It is important for us to be respectful of and live by these rhythms. When God created everything He said it is all very good. He created these rhythms and if we ignore His plans long enough, we will pay and the domino effect will take place! We must make a choice; yes a choice of how we want to live. If we really want to be fruitful, then we need to figure out how to balance life, work, and leisure.

Symptoms of Sleep Deprivation

Following are some of the symptoms of sleep deprivation and in order of their occurrence from least severe to the worst:

1. General Fatigue

An overall feeling of lack of energy and fatigue

2. Emotional Irritability

Depression, irritability, anger, frustration, anxiety

3. Cognitive Impairment

Reduced capacity for intellectual acuity

4. Physical Impairment

Decreased reaction time, diminished muscle strength, and decreased cardio   endurance.

5. Psychosis

Emotionally unstable, unrealistic, hearing voices, seeing weird things, and so forth

6. Death...

Any animal will at some point die if they do not get sleep.

Chronic sleep deprivation has been linked to high blood pressure, cancer, heart disease, diabetes, and obesity. Sleep helps maintain a healthy balance of the hormones that make you feel hungry (ghrelin) or full (leptin). When you do not get enough sleep, your level of ghrelin goes up and your level of leptin goes down. This makes you feel hungrier than when you are well rested.

Lack of sleep affects your reaction to insulin, the hormone that controls your blood glucose (sugar) level. Lack of sleep encourages a higher than normal blood sugar level and that can increase you risk for diabetes.

Sleep also supports healthy growth and development. Deep sleep triggers the body to release the hormone that promotes normal growth in children and teens. That same hormone also supports muscle mass and helps repair cells and tissues in children, teens, and adults.

Your immune system relies on sleep to stay healthy. Your immune system fights off unhealthy organisms that want to invade your body. Ongoing sleep deficiency can change the way in which your immune system responds. For example, if you are sleep deficient, you may have trouble fighting common infections like colds and flu.

Most people, hopefully, will never experience the more severe and dangerous side effects of lack of sleep. Nonetheless, many will go through life tired and crabby. Lacking energy to remember birthdays, or to send messages, make phone calls or even have the spirit to tell jokes or take healthy risks and be adventurous, fostering meaningful relationships will be difficult. And, instead of being Christians that are a fountain of joy, these people will just be completely pooped! The worst part is these people can be so entirely exhausted they just do not care about anything!

A Biblical Perspective about Sleep and Rest

Jesus invites people:

Matthew 11: 28– 29 (NIV)

"Come to me, all you who are weary and burdened, and I will give you rest. Take my yoke upon you and learn from me, for I am gentle and humble in heart, and you will find rest for your souls."

Jesus died on the cross to bring peace. And rest. And wellness.

Benefits of Enough Sleep

- **Improves Memory**
- **Prolongs Life**
- **Less Inflammation.** People who get less than six hours of sleep a night have higher levels of inflammatory proteins than those who get more sleep. A study done in 2010 showed that C-reactive protein, which is associated with heart attack risk, was higher in the people who got six or less hours of sleep a night. Inflammation is also linked to stroke, diabetes, arthritis, and premature aging.

123

- **Boosts Creativity**
- **Improves Physical Performance.** A study done on college football players showed their average sprint time improved when they got at least 10 hours of sleep a night for seven to eight weeks. And, their day-time fatigue was decreased and their overall stamina was increased.
- **Increases Learning.** If you have big reports to get done or tests to take or anything that requires intellectual information to be processed, sleep makes a huge difference.
- **Sharpens Attention.** Lack of sleep in children around seven or eight years old will actually result in ADHD type behaviors. If they got less than eight hours of sleep they were more likely to be hyperactive, inattentive, and impulsive.
- **Promotes Healthy Weight.** Well- rested people lose more fat than those who are sleep-deprived. Also, adequate sleep decreases the appetite and loss of sleep makes you feel hungrier.
- **Lowers Stress.** Sleep can lower your stress which lowers your blood pressure. It is also widely believed that good sleep has an effect on cholesterol levels, which has a lot to do with heart disease

- **Lowers Risk of Accidents.** Lack of sleep for just one night can be as bad on your driving as having an alcoholic drink!
- **Reduce Depression**. Good sleep can help a moody person lower their anxiety and grumpy attitude.

How to Sleep Better

- Keep a regular sleep and wake schedule.
- Do not drink or eat caffeine four to six hours before bed and minimize daytime use.

Rest is a necessity. It is a Biblical principle that all creatures must rest. Without proper rest the human body will break down.

- Do not smoke – especially near bedtime or if you wake up in the night
- Avoid alcohol and heavy meals before sleep.
- Get regular exercise.
- Minimize noise, light, and excessive hot and cold temperatures where you sleep,
- Develop a regular bed time and go to bed at the same time each night,
- Try to wake up without an alarm clock,
- Attempt to go to bed earlier every night for certain period; this will ensure that you are getting enough sleep.

 125

This is a very good video clip of Dr. Oz discussing how lack of sleep affects us. The first seven minutes of the video cover the sleep topic. The rest of the video is about other topics. When you have a chance, go to this website and listen to what he has to say. You might be surprised at what you hear! Here is the link: http://www.youtube.com/watch?v=LH-pYQ7X85s

How to Recognize Sleep Deprivation in Yourself and Others

This is a fun little game on line that tests your reaction time. Play the game twice – first, when you are well rested, and then when you are very tired. It is amazing what happens. When I took it the second time, I thought I was well rested, but my score made it look like I was well, under the influence! After all, one night of less than adequate sleep is equivalent to driving with one alcoholic beverage in your system. Here is the link. It is fun, enlightening, and worthwhile. http://healthysleep.med.harvard.edu/need-sleep/whats-in-it-for-you/how-awake-are-you

In this video clip, Dr. Mercola gives you all kinds of sleep tips. He makes some very good points and I think you will hear some suggestions you have never heard before.

It is about nine minutes long. Here is the link: http://www.youtube.com/watch?v=gwwe5Zis6VI

Bible Verses about Sleep and Rest

Rest is a necessity. It is a Biblical principle that all creatures must rest. Without proper rest the human body will break down. I know I have had a good night's rest when I wake up refreshed and rejuvenated. Take a look at what the Bible says about rest:

Genesis 2:2-3 (NIV)

"By the seventh day God had finished the work he had been doing; so on the seventh day he rested from all his work. ³ Then God blessed the seventh day and made it holy, because on it he rested from all the work of creating that he had done."

Exodus 20:8-10 (NIV)

"Remember the Sabbath day by keeping it holy. Six days you shall labor and do all your work, but the seventh day is a Sabbath to the LORD your God. On it you shall not do any work, neither you, nor your son or daughter, nor your male or female servant, nor your animals, nor any foreigner residing in your towns."

Exodus 23:12 (NIV)

"Six days do your work, but on the seventh day do not work, so that your ox and your donkey may rest, and so that the slave born in your household and the foreigner living among you may be refreshed."

God Grants Rest Not Only for Man
Genesis 8:4 (NIV)

"and on the seventeenth day of the seventh month the ark came to rest on the mountains of Ararat.

Song of Solomon 1:7 (MSG)

"Tell me where you're working—I love you so much— Tell me where you're tending your flocks, where you let them rest at noontime. Why should I be the one left out, outside the orbit of your tender care?"

Jeremiah 33:12 (NIV)

"This is what the LORD Almighty says: 'In this place, desolate and without people or animals—in all its towns there will again be pastures for shepherds to rest their flocks.

God Provides Rest from Trouble

Psalms 37:7 (NIV)

Be still before the LORD and wait patiently for him;
do not fret when people succeed in their ways,
when they carry out their wicked schemes.

Psalms 55:6 (NIV)

*I said, "Oh, that I had the wings of a dove! I would
fly away and be at rest.*

Isaiah 14:3-4 (NIV)

*"On the day the LORD gives you relief from your
suffering and turmoil and from the harsh labor
forced on you, you will take up this taunt against the
king of Babylon: How the oppressor has come to an
end! How his fury has ended!"*

God Promises Rest and Peace from Anxiety

Ecclesiastes 2:24-25 (NIV)

*"A person can do nothing better than to eat and
drink and find satisfaction in their own toil. This
too, I see, is from the hand of God, for without him,
who can eat or find enjoyment?"*

2 Corinthians 2:13-14 (NIV)

"I still had no peace of mind, because I did not find my brother Titus there. So I said goodbye to them and went on to Macedonia. But thanks be to God, who always leads us as captives in Christ's triumphal procession and uses us to spread the aroma of the knowledge of him everywhere."

Philippians 4:6-7 (NIV)

"Do not be anxious about anything, but in every situation, by prayer and petition, with thanksgiving, present your requests to God. And the peace of God, which transcends all understanding, will guard your hearts and your minds in Christ Jesus."

God Knows You Must Rest to Recuperate; Even in Ministry

Mark 6:31 (NIV)

"Do not be anxious about anything, but in every situation, by prayer and petition, with thanksgiving, present your requests to God. And the peace of God, which transcends all understanding, will guard your hearts and your minds in Christ Jesus."

Matthew 8:24(NIV)

"Suddenly a furious storm came up on the lake, so that the waves swept over the boat. But Jesus was sleeping. (Jesus rested)"

Matthew 26:45 (NIV)

"Then he returned to the disciples and said to them, "Are you still sleeping and resting? Look, the hour has come, and the Son of Man is delivered into the hands of sinners."

God Gives Spiritual Rest for the Soul

Jeremiah 6:16 (NIV)

"This is what the LORD says: "Stand at the crossroads and look; ask for the ancient paths, ask where the good way is, and walk in it, and you will find rest for your souls. But you said, 'We will not walk in it.'"

Matthew 11:28-29 (NIV)

"...Come to me, all you who are weary and burdened, and I will give you rest. Take my yoke

upon you and learn from me, for I am gentle and humble in heart, and you will find rest for your souls."

Hebrews 4:4; 9-10 (NIV)

"For somewhere he has spoken about the seventh day in these words: "On the seventh day God rested from all his works. There remains, then, a Sabbath-rest for the people of God; for anyone who enters God's rest also rests from their works, just as God did from his"

Revelation 6:11 (NIV)

"Then each of them was given a white robe, and they were told to wait a little longer, until the full number of their fellow servants, their brothers and sisters, were killed just as they had been."

Revelation 14:13 (NIV)

"Then I heard a voice from heaven say, "Write this: Blessed are the dead who die in the Lord from now on." "Yes," says the Spirit, "they will rest from their labor, for their deeds will follow them."

I found most of these verses at this website http://www.whatchristianswanttoknow.com/ They have many more if you want to gather more for your use.

So, go and get your rest so you can get ready to absorb the next chapter!

Chapter 6: Relationships

People have said on their death beds that the only thing that really matters in life is your family and friends. In other words, your relationships are the most important things in life.

The bible says we are to work hard at living in peace with others (1 Peter 3:11).

Brian Hathaway has estimated that 44% of the letters of the New Testament are about how we should get along with one another. This contrasts with about 4% on spiritual gifts. I do not know about you, but I am led to conclude that much of our teaching should deal with relationships. And, all of our relationships begin with our relationship with God.

When our relationship with God is strong and thriving, the Holy Spirit grows various qualities in us know as the fruit of the Spirit.

Galatians 5:22-23 (NIV)

"But the fruit of the Spirit is love, joy, peace, forbearance, kindness, goodness, faithfulness, gentleness and self-control. Against such things there is no law."

How does this fruit help us work toward unity in our relationships? A healthy relationship produces love, joy, peace, patience, kindness, goodness, faithfulness, gentleness, and self-control.

God is almighty in every aspect of our lives. He came through Jesus Christ and demonstrated and told us everything we need to know to live a life of happiness, abundance, and fulfillment.

Jesus started working with relationships since He was little. He spent much of his time conversing, exchanging, and interpreting ideas and God's word. Then He demonstrated love and discipline in the wilderness overcoming the greatest temptations on earth. That was His preparation for beginning to show His glory and love for us and pay in whole for any sin we have committed and will commit on earth.

In my opinion, the three greatest lessons for anyone who wants live a life of happiness, abundance, and fulfillment are:

1. Love God and only God.

2. Love your neighbor as yourself!

3. Treat others the way you want to be treated!

Most of us have no issue loving God, but we falter when it comes to loving others and ourselves. Once we can learn to love ourselves, we can accept and love others too. When you understand what is involved in accepting and loving yourself, then you can begin to understand others and their uniqueness.

Making investments into any relationship account is done with courtesy, kindness, honesty, and keeping commitments.

You know that long-lasting relationships have no shortcuts. Many people are desperately trying to get into a loving relationship before they learn to accept and love themselves, and it does not work. If you cannot take care of and love yourself, you will not have any idea or strength to care for anyone else either.

Causes for Relationship Break Downs

God created Adam and Adam had a great relationship with God and all of His creation. Then, God, knowing Adam had a deeper need for a companion "like him," created Eve. Oh, how fulfilled Adam and Eve were with this beautiful relationship. They knew of no ugliness, arguments, or disharmony because they were walking daily with God and in accordance with His will.

God provided them with everything they needed and told them there was only one thing in the garden they could not have. He told them not eat of the tree of the knowledge of good and evil as it would bring death. Then, the serpent came along and convinced Eve to just taste that amazing fruit, who in turn did the same with Adam. Suddenly their whole world

You know that long-lasting relationships have no shortcuts.
Many people are desperately trying to get into a loving relationship before they learn to accept and love themselves, and it does not work.

changed. There was fear! They had never experienced fear before and now they were afraid of what God would say and do. They became irresponsible and when God asked them about this event, Adam blamed Eve and Eve blamed the serpent. No one took responsibility for their actions. It spoiled their relationship with God and with each other.

We all have specific, fear at our core. Do you suppose Adam and Eve felt the core fear of disconnection from God? Fear - He would no longer listen to, value, or love them? Did they fear

137

being helpless?   Did they fear being a failure, rejected, abandoned, defective, inadequate, manipulated, or isolated?

So go our relationships today. All is going well until someone or something happens that hurts or causes fear in the other and then it is everyone else's fault! Responsibility goes by the wayside and is replaced with pointing fingers. Here is how fear might look in the context of our culture:

1. **Something happens in a relationship to cause pain.**

    Pain might even be caused by something meant to be a kind gesture, but the other person felt devalued by it. For example: You have a friend who may be going through financial hardships. You buy your friend a few groceries and drop them by the house. You are thinking this was a really nice thing to do and you feel good because you are helping, but your friend gets upset because she feels devalued, worthless, and a failure.

2. **Fear shows up and crazy reactions happen**

    Your friend starts complaining about what you bought. She does not like the brand you bought. Her kids will not eat broccoli – you should have known they only eat green beans.   She begins to react to your generosity negatively because of her fear of being a worthless failure. She even gets a little smug and starts to devalue you because you should have known what she really needed. Before you know it, she in a full-blown rant about all kinds of issues in the past. Of course, none of this has anything to do with groceries or the past!

3. Then you are hurt and want your needs met

You just wanted to help! All you wanted was a little appreciation! How ungrateful your friend is! Now you are afraid that your friend will no longer love and value you and your friendship. Now it is your turn to feel like a failure. You beat yourself up because your friend was right. You really should have known better. I am a terrible friend. I hurt my friend deeply. What was I thinking? I am no good to anyone?

4. Now you react

So now you begin to yell at your friend and tell her how ungrateful she is. You were just trying to help and now she is making a big deal out of your attempt to befriend her in a time of need. You take the groceries back and say you will just give them to the next person you see on the street. They will be far more thankful that your friend was, and you leave in a huff!

5. **And on and on it goes, repeating itself over and over again**

   How do we stop this cycle? Take personal responsibility!
   These are the two ways to succeed in relationships.

   1. You must take care of yourself and be at your best
      physically, mentally, emotionally, and spiritually.

   2. Empower everyone you meet with care, open
      communication, and positive interaction.

Learning to manage your feelings is accepting responsibility to manage your relationships. Think of your relationships like this: you have a "relationship account" with each one of them. In this account, you make deposits and withdrawals. You build a reserve with positive and empowering communication. And you make withdrawals with negative moments that subtract from your reserve.

The relationship account will let you know how to act with and respond to the other person. You will want to build a huge reserve of trust in relationships. Your account will let you know how free or careful you must be with that person.

Making investments into any relationship account is done with courtesy, kindness, honesty, and keeping

People have said on their death bed that the only thing that really matters in life is your family and friends. In other words, your relationships throughout your life are the most important things in life.

commitments. If you build up a reserve and raise the trust on the account, you will be allowed to speak into this person's life and will give them permission or status to do the same for you. You know you can call on this person whenever you need something and they can do the same with you. This is a healthy relationship.

A high reserve gives you a margin of error in the relationship. You trust each other's hearts. Communication does not even need to be completely clear. You understand each other when your trust account balance is high and communication becomes easier. Conversely, if you are typically discourteous, disrespectful, foolishly kidding, ignoring, or betraying trust your relationship account will become empty or even run a deficit. If your trust is wiped out, you have no room for error. You are walking around gingerly, like you are crossing a land mine field. Now you must be very careful with what you say, because every word will be measured.

The result of this dynamic is living in tension. Sometimes people abandon face-to-face interaction for fear of misinterpretation, and choose to communicate via email, notes, and memos.

When a couple does not keep a large reserve of trust in the account, their marriage breaks down. The communication goes from being spontaneous to carefully crafted words. These individuals begin to adapt by living separately together. Of course this does not work, so communication becomes hostile and defensive. The resulting arguments make relating too difficult, so now they just stop talking altogether.

It is sad. Two individuals came together from a very close and loving relationship and now each of them sees the other as the last person with whom they want to spend time.

All relationships need to build reserve accounts. But marriages are especially important, as this relationship has long-term and ongoing expectations for relationship health. This is entirely different than seeing an old friend whom you have not seen for years. It is awesome when you pick up right where you left off years ago! The deposits are still there from the last time you saw them. Hopefully when things get tense in a marriage, each person can draw on the same kind of reserve that was in place before they were married.

Three Things You Must Know about Relationships

1. There are no quick fixes

2. Building and repairing are long-term investments

3. You cannot keep pulling up the flowers to see how the roots are growing

Six Effective Deposits to Build Any Relationship

1. Understand the Individual

To make a true deposit, you must put value on what the other person says and value the things he or she values. You do not have to agree with what the other says, but you need to respect the opinion of the other by paying close attention to what is said and the feeling behind the words.

One of my friends wanted to get closer to his son so he became intensely involved in tennis because that was his son's favorite sport. He followed his son to tournaments every week for an entire summer. I asked my friend, "Do you like tennis that much?" "No," he replied, "but I love my son that much."

Remember this little story the next time you want to build your relationship account. Instead of doing the things we would like, think about what the other person would like.

2. Pay Attention to the Little Things

Any discourtesy, unkindness, and disrespect make huge withdrawals in the personal relationships account. In close relationships, it is the little things that become huge. We expect much more from those closest to us.

Consider your relationships: How happy are you? How strong are you in listening and understanding? How quickly do you turn on the people closest to you?

When your account is high, you feel positive and good towards those you love. But if that person makes a mistake, hopefully there will still be enough in reserve for you to continue to accept that person.

When reserves are high, you are able to laugh off the times you accidentally step on each other's toes – literally and figuratively. But when your account is near zero balance, reactions take the form of nasty remarks, disapproving looks, and such. Being truly close and vulnerable with others puts us in the position where we can step on each other's toes or accidentally trip each other up. This is why it is so important for you to work on keeping your relationship accounts high.

3. Keep Commitments

Keeping a commitment or a promise is a big deposit, but breaking one is a huge withdrawal. In fact, I think the biggest withdrawal someone can make is to break a promise because next time, they will not trust you! Do not ever make a promise you cannot keep. Learn to make promises very carefully, checking out anything that could prevent you from fulfilling it. However, when a situation makes it impossible for you to keep a promise, you must find a true course of apologizing.

4. Clarify Expectations

It is very important to have clear expectations in a relationship. Functioning on assumptions gets us all into trouble. We need to sit down with each other periodically to discuss and define our roles and expectations of each other so that we can operate clearly and be able to make a lot of deposits in each other's relationship account. When we operate on assumptions, we might as well just pull the plug on our relationships account as we will be making mistake after mistake assuming we know what is expected. This can be the demise of many relationships, and quickly!

5. Personal Integrity

Personal integrity generates trust and as a result, large deposits in a relationship account. However, lack of integrity undermines trust and results in many withdrawals from the account.

Integrity is being loyal to those not present, which will build the trust with those present. When you defend the absent, you create trust of the present. Integrity is consistently treating everyone with the same set of principles. This creates trust. Your honesty may make people feel uncomfortable at first, but they will honor you in the end.

To confront others takes a lot more courage. However, most people prefer the course of least resistance and opt to belittle, criticize, betray confidences, or gossip about others. People trust and respect you when you are honest and clear with them. If you have the courage to face others with integrity, you will be trusted. Trust comes first and love is right behind it. Integrity avoids deceptive communication.

6. Apologize When Making a Withdrawal

Anytime you make withdrawals from the relationship account, apologize sincerely. When you apologize, you can keep your deposits in that account if you use phrases such as: "I did wrong." - "That was not nice of me." - "I lacked respect." "I ignored you, and I am very sorry." - "I had no right to embarrass you in front of your friends. I apologize."

You need to be internally strong to apologize from the heart. Only people with internal security can apologize with sincerity. People with little internal security cannot do it, they are too weak, and they would be afraid to be taken advantage of. This kind of person's security comes from the opinions of others and they would worry about what others think of them and therefore their apology would not be heartfelt.

Leo Roskin said: "It's the weak who are cruel. Gentleness can only come from the strong." Sincere apologies make good deposits in the account; insincere and repeated apologies become withdrawals, and the relationship will show it.

Ways to Keep Your Relationship Account High in Marriage

Remember that all things count, so be courteous and show your appreciation of what your partner means to you and brings into your life. Be attentive to, supportive p, and genuinely interested in your partner.

Do something special. Go out of your way for your partner. Think about what's important to your partner and follow through with a loving gesture. Have respectful discussions. All couples have disagreements, so when you do, always keep your communication respectful. Do not judge the other person, and resist the urge to make your perception correct.

Think in terms of your relationship account, and gauge the strength of your relationships. If your account is getting down close to zero, start making positive deposits. It's not wise to wait for that to happen. The best caring strategy in any relationship is to always make regular deposits and maintain healthy relationships.

How Does this Look from a Coaching Aspect?

The Wellness Coaching Course (www.pccca.org/wellness) expands significantly on the following points.

I love this verse as it describes a strong characteristic of a great coach.

Proverbs 29:5 (NIV)

"Those who flatter their neighbors are spreading nets for their feet."

Another translation says, "if you are smart, you will draw it out." Being a good relationships coach means you have to be able to draw things out of your clients by asking those thought-provoking questions. Many people having relationship issues need you to help them verbalize their feelings by drawing out their thoughts, piece-by-piece in order to help them put it all together.

Relationship coaching can involve a wide array of issues. Here are a few for you to ponder and consider where your strengths as a coach may be. You will also want to assess what additional education you may need in order to be an effective relationship coach.

Many of your clients may suffer from overload or burnout as a result of unhealthy relationships. The source of could be work, family, friends and other life relationships in general. Some will come to you because they long for a meaningful relationship with God. They want to be closer to their Creator and just cannot find that path to get there. You may find that when dealing with a client's relationship issues, it may boil down to having a meaningful relationship with God that will make a difference in the original issue. As you can see, wellness coaching does not take place in a vacuum. One type of coaching can easily lead to other, related issues.

Some people are simply searching for meaning and purpose.

Many are looking for the deep meaning behind why a partner, friend, coworker, or family member behaves in a particular way. Sometimes the client is trying to understand the role he or she plays in that relationship.

Sometimes people feel lonely even though they are in a relationship. Not all relationships are fulfilling. Some relationships are shallow, lacking in intimacy and meaning. The absence of meaningful relationships can lead to anxiety and depression. Also, meaningful relationships are oftentimes built on common interests. When a couple can no longer identify anything in common, the relationship will suffer. In today's age of technology and automation, deep relationships are not as prevalent as they once were. Face-to-face conversation is going away in place of email, texting, computer technology, and lack of time!

Being a parent is a relationship that can leave people overwhelmed and inadequate. If you have raised children, you already know the heartaches, battles, and joys that come with parenting. Parents do not often think about how they can end up feeling lonely in their role. Sometimes it seems nothing goes right, but as the one responsible for raising healthy children, parents may be reluctant to admit need for emotional support.

When marriages do not live up to the idealist expectations of a couple, they may seek relationship coaching. Depending on the couple, this is a prime example of where counseling may be more appropriate before coaching begins. As a coach, you are responsible for knowing the limitations of your skills. If you have any doubt about your ability to help, you should promptly refer them to someone better equipped to help them at this stage, keeping the door open for when coaching is more appropriate.

Dr. Bush has an amazing course on relationships (http://speaklove.weebly.com/) that you will find helpful in dealing with this topic. Some people like to specialize in this area and find her program is very beneficial to their business.

I would like to draw this chapter to a close with this sweet story that to me depicts the "character" of a truly beautiful relationship. Inspirational Quotes - Pictures - Motivational Thoughts http://rishikajain.com/2013/01/08heart-touching-beautiful-story-a-very-poor--man/

A very poor man lived with his wife. One day his wife, who had very long hair, asked him to buy her a comb for her hair to grow well and to be well-groomed. The man felt very sorry and said no. He explained that he did not even have enough money to fix the strap of his watch he had just broken. She did not insist on her request. The man went to work and passed by a watch shop, sold his damaged watch at a low price and went to buy a comb for his wife. He came home in the evening with the comb in his hand, ready to give to his wife. He was surprised when he saw his wife with a very short hair cut. She had sold her hair and was holding a new watch band. Tears flowed simultaneously from their eyes, not for the futility of their actions, but for the reciprocity of their love.

Moral: To love is nothing, to be loved is something, but to love and to be loved by the one you love, that is everything. Never take love for granted.

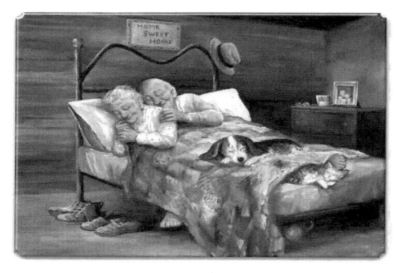

Now that's a healthy relationship! Ah, so sweet!

Chapter 7: Natural Wellness

Leelo Bush, Ph.D.

The information contained in this chapter is for informational purposes only. The contents are not intended to provide a professional medical diagnosis, opinion or to recommend any particular course of treatment.

Our health and well-being are important to God. His word urges us to take responsibility for our own health-related decisions. Our first job is to learn about our body and how it works. Then we need to learn what is naturally available to help us. Pharmaceuticals have a place in health care, and so do natural medicines. We need to become and remain proactive in seeking optimum health and wellness.

Over two thousand years ago, the Christ child received gifts of frankincense and myrrh, two highly valued essential oils. Today these oils and others are available to you in their purest form. If they were good enough for Jesus, should they not be good enough for us? Let us begin to explore this viable option more in depth.

Take Good Care of Your Temple!

Get plenty of rest. Eat a balanced diet of natural foods, rather than reconstituted foods. Exercise regularly and ask our healthcare professional any time you need a medical opinion.

Live with hope and expectancy. God has a great plan for you!

I did not know, what I did not know.

As I look back now, it is incredible to me I did not know anything about God's provision for our healing. In my naiveté, I believed medicine began with modern medical science and antibiotics. I can hardly believe how much I had missed. While I made a decision long ago to become responsible for my own health and well-being, I had not been exposed to other viable alternatives.

Please do not feel badly if you have bought into modern medicine and related philosophies as I did. If you believe the best healing always happens as a result of strategies provided by your medical doctor (M.D.), then you are like 80% or more Americans. It may surprise you to learn though, that likely 80% of the rest of the world has access to and gives credence to natural, God-created solutions.

Regardless of access to western healthcare, there may be times when you look for alternatives: maybe as a first line of defense or perhaps if other solutions are not working as needed. It is my hope that this information triggers further research and discovery for you and your health.

Natural solutions are, in their optimum form, plant-based and pure, without any chemicals, petroleum derivatives or pollutants. They contain nothing man-made, which could affect their efficacy, potency, or cause our immune system to reject

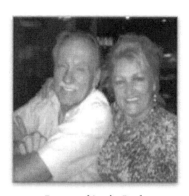

Evan and Leelo Bush

them. Indeed, the pure, essential oils from plants were created by the same author who intelligently designed each cell of our being. It should be no surprise then, that the gift of nature would be most compatible with our human physiology as well as with the physiology of other animals, all of whom are God's handiwork.

With that said, it is of critical importance that essential oils be pure. Only one company that I am aware of at this writing has externally-tested and certified pure, therapeutic grade essential oils. That company is dōTERRA and you will see me refer to them time and time again.

The information in this chapter is neither complete nor is it written to answer every question and offer a remedy for every ailment. Instead, I have added it so you may be more informed and have a basis for further research. Other books do this much better than I could with the space allotted. At the end of this chapter, I will offer you web resources so you can obtain further information, training, products, and discounts if you would like to try them.

How I Discovered Essential Oils

In 2012, I had been ill for several months, having lost my voice with flu-like symptoms. After numerous visits to my doctor (MD), and after four courses of various antibiotics, I was still not healthy. I would begin to improve for a day or two and then be right back where I started. Being a teacher and speaker, with our annual Christian Life Coach and Counselor conference, the Barefoot Mastermind (www.barefootmastermind.com) approaching, I was very concerned. I needed my voice but more than that, I needed to be well.

Meanwhile, my husband, Evan, had been experiencing a lot of pain in his legs and knees. Thousand-dollar shots at the doctor's office were out of the question because our insurance did not cover them. My massage therapist suggested I give him a drop of *Deep Blue*® essential oil on each knee and see whether he experiences any benefit. We tried this one evening and the next morning he arose from bed with almost no pain at all. He stayed the course with treating his legs with a few drops of oil as needed until a month later, he was completely healthy again.

I knew I had to know more about what worked so well for him, so when my massage therapist invited us to a class about the oils, I felt compelled to attend and took Evan with me. While at this two-hour class, I likely tried 20 various essential oils and heard stories of others' healing as well. I had no inkling what to expect but I could feel later that evening something was going on inside me. I had used many of the oils and felt a bit "tingly", for lack of better description. The next morning I awoke completely well and I have not been ill since. Now at the first sign of a cold, stomach upset or flu, I reach for an essential oil.

The "Science" Behind what Probably Happened in our Healing

We learned in class that many physical complaints arise as a result of inflammation. Injury and toxicity can cause inflammation. When *Deep Blue*® relieved the inflammation in Evan's legs, natural healing could occur from the inside out.

Over time I also learned that essential oils can destroy not only harmful bacteria and fungus, but also viruses in our bodies.

Antibiotics only help against bacteria. It is likely I had a virus that antibiotics could not touch, yet the essential oil was effective.

Essential oils can destroy not only harmful bacteria and fungus but also viruses in our bodies. Antibiotics only help against bacteria

You see, antibiotics kill bacteria outside our cells. So, if there is a virus inside our cell, the antibiotic is of no help. However an essential oil with antiviral properties can penetrate the cell membrane and heal the cell from the inside out. Then it continues to protect the newly healthy cells, boosting our immune system.

Unlike antibiotics, certified pure therapeutic grade (CPTG) oils are pure and designed by God to work with our systems. As a result, we do not develop an intolerance or immunity to them.

That said, we must become knowledgeable about which oils to use and how to use them. Some oils can be taken internally, some topically and some used aromatically. Because of their potency, some people (particularly when caring for a child), may find they need to dilute the essential oil with a carrier oil such as coconut, olive or vegetable oil.

If you are new to essential oil therapy, then allow me to give you a quick explanation.

The following can be found on the dōTERRA site: "Essential oils are natural, aromatic compounds found in the seeds, bark, stems, flowers, roots, and other parts of plants. They can be both beautifully and powerfully fragrant. If you have ever enjoyed the gift of a rose, a walk by a field of lavender, or the smell of fresh cut mint, you have experienced the aromatic qualities of essential oils. In addition to giving plants their distinctive smells, essential oils provide plants with protection against predators and disease and play a role in plant pollination.

Essential oils are non-water-based phytochemicals made up of volatile, organic compounds. Although they are fat soluble, they do not include fatty lipids or acids found in vegetable and animal oils. Essential oils are very clean, almost crisp to the touch and are immediately absorbed by the skin. Pure, unadulterated essential oils are translucent and range in color from crystal clear to deep blue.

Try this at home: Squeeze the peel of a ripe orange. The fragrant residue on your hand is full of essential oils. In addition to their intrinsic benefits to plants and being beautifully fragrant to people, essential oils have been used throughout history in many cultures for their medicinal and therapeutic benefits. Modern scientific study and trends towards more holistic approaches to wellness are driving a revival and new discovery of essential oil health applications.

CAUTION – Verify Oil Grade before Using!

(Excerpt from Dr. Matt Hale)

Caution: Before you rub any oil onto your skin or take it internally, first find out what really is in the oil, where it was sourced from and how it was created.

SYNTHETIC – PERFUME & INDUSTRIAL GRADE - The lowest level of quality is what is put in our perfumes. These are usually synthetic with all the compounds being synthetic.

USED IN FOOD – G.R.A.S. STANDARD - The second lowest level of quality of essential oils is used in foods. These have to abide by the generally-regarded-as-safe (G.R.A.S.) standard. These oils are used as flavor substitutes or flavor enhancers.

THERAPEUTIC – HAVE HEALTH BENEFIT - The next level is therapeutic grade. This level of essential oil is what massage therapists and natural healers use. When an oil is therapeutic grade, the manufacturer is legally allowed to put 100% pure on the bottle. In order for an oil to be labeled 100% pure, it must be tested by a gas chromatograph test. This test looks at the compounds that make up the oil to see if they are all there. If the oil passes, then the manufacturer can label it 100% pure. However, there are three problems with the gas chromatograph test:

It should be no surprise then, that essential oils, our gift of nature, would be most compatible with our human physiology as well as with the physiology of other animals, all of whom are God's handiwork.

1. The test does not check for foreign impurities. In other words, weeds harvested with the essential oil plant, pesticides, or anything extra that should not be there may very well be there.

2. The test does not check for exact amounts of the compounds that should be in the oil. As long as they are all there, the oil gets a stamp of approval.

3. The test does not assess whether or not the compounds are 100% natural or if they are synthetic.

Note: *An essential oil could have every single compound required to be labeled as 100% pure, even if all compounds are synthetic.* The gas chromatograph test is an industry standard but clearly not a sufficient way of testing by itself. dōTERRA believed there should be a higher standard for testing to ensure oils people are using are really 100% pure and synthetic-free.

TOP GRADE – CERTIFIED PURE THERAPEUTIC GRADE (CPTG) - The highest grade of essential oils.

To accomplish this dōTERRA created a new standard called Certified Pure Therapeutic Grade or CPTG for short. For an oil to receive this certification it must also go through a mass spectrometry test. This test checks to make sure no foreign impurities are in the oil. It not only checks to make sure the oil has the correct compounds in the exact amounts, but it absolutely identifies if the oil or any part of it is synthetic in any way.

Most companies do not do the mass spectrometry test or they do it infrequently. Some do it in-house. However, dōTERRA uses an independent lab, a third party, and checks every vial of every batch to make sure consumers receive the same pure oil each time.

dōTERRA (meaning "Gift of the Earth") essential oils represent the safest, purest essential oils available in the world today.

As a side note; dōTERRA oils also go through the following additional testing:

- Arganoleptic evaluation: appearance of the oil -- does it look like it is supposed to?
- Microbiological evaluation: Tests for presences of any bacteria such as coliform or salmonella
- Shelf life testing
- Heavy metal testing
- FT-IR (infrared technology): Fingerprint of the oil

dōTERRA oils must pass rigorous testing before ever being offered to the consumers. This is the mark of true CPTG oil.

Note: *Each essential oil can have from 50 – 200+ compounds that make up the oil. Each compound helps with different things in your body. To give you an idea of how many that is, an antibiotic you would get from your doctor would be made up of 2-4 compounds.*

Scriptures that refer to oils in the Bible:

Exodus 30:22-25 (NIV)

"Then the LORD said to Moses ,"Take the following fine spices: 500 shekels[a] of liquid myrrh, half as much (that is, 250 shekels) of fragrant cinnamon, 250 shekels of fragrant calamus, 500 shekels of cassia—all according to the sanctuary shekel—and a hin of olive oil. Make these into a sacred anointing oil, a fragrant blend, the work of a perfumer. It will be the sacred anointing oil."

(For additional references, see: http://livinganointed.com/testimonials/bible-references.html)

In his book, *Healing Oils of the Bible*, by David Stewart, Ph.D., the author lists over 500 biblical references to essential oils, aromatic plants, and their uses. The book is both scriptural and scientific and its premise is that healing is a sacred art, rather than a secular science. For those interested in more

Squeeze the peel of a ripe orange. The fragrant residue on your hand is full of essential oils.

in-depth knowledge on this topic, Stewart's book contains notes on how you can do a Bible oils program in your community.

Essential Oils in the Bible

(http://www.godsforgottengift.com/oils.shtml)

We read in the first chapter of Genesis that God placed mankind in the Garden of Eden. God knew from the very beginning that this perfect environment would be the key source for mankind's healing and health.

Daily applications of essential oils in biblical times were extensive, indeed. Thirty-six of the 39 books of the Old Testament and 10 of the 27 books of the New Testament mention essential oils or the plants that produce them. These oils are the medicine provided by God.

The early Christians held the aromatic oils in very high esteem. Paul chose to compare devout Christians as "sweet savors," "fragrances," or "aromas" spreading the Gospel "among the perishing." In Ephesians 5:2, he encourages his fellow Christians to be imitators of Christ "who gave himself up for us, as a fragrant offering and sacrifice to God."

God provided these plants and oils to heal our bodies, minds, and spirits. They were the original source of healing and that connection is still available to us today. "Healing: God's Forgotten Gift" is meant to be a guide to help us all to explore and learn what tools God make available to us to help keep us healthy physically, emotionally and spiritually.

Dr. Matt Hale writes: "I remember being a young child and asking someone at church why the wise men gave the baby Jesus frankincense and myrrh. Gold seemed to make sense. I mean, who would not want that? But the other two, I just didn't quite get. The response was unsatisfying but became my reality for the next 30 years. 'They were very valuable, sweetie,' I was told. 'They just wanted to give Him something very valuable because He is very valuable.'"

I have been around scripture too long to continue to accept a superficial answer. I am forever surprised at the level of symbolism that exists if we are willing to dig. Recently I was asked to speak on the balms of the scriptures -- specifically the Balm of Gilead. This is where I found my answer. A balm is a medicinal compound of essential oils, resin, and sometimes other plant material. Balms have been around for thousands of years and can still be used today to naturally heal wounds and promote health. A significant component of the Balm of Gilead was most likely derived from myrrh resin. While during my research it dawned on me that myrrh and frankincense are both taken from a tree. Specifically, the tree is wounded and bleeds.

This resin is then taken and used to heal wounds. The Savior is the Tree of Life.

Revelation 2:7 (NIV)

"Whoever has ears, let them hear what the Spirit says to the churches. To the one who is victorious, I will give the right to eat from the tree of life, which is in the paradise of God."

Acts 5:30 (NIV)

"The God of our ancestors raised Jesus from the dead—whom you killed by hanging him on a cross."

At that moment I realized that both frankincense and myrrh represent the Savior. But that is only the beginning. The gifts were given by men from the east. We do not know exactly where, but we do know that it was far enough away that they were not part of the Hebrew culture. So the golden question is: What did people from the east believe about frankincense and myrrh?

Frankincense was used in the Jewish temples as spiritual incense. Frankincense represents our spirits and specifically represents the balm of our spirits, representing Christ as the balm of our spiritual wounds.

In eastern medicine <u>myrrh</u> was used to stimulate the heart, liver, and spleen. But, it was by far most recognized for its ability to circulate stagnant blood. Blood represents mortality. Myrrh was used by the Jews to anoint women before and after child birth.

Myrrh then represents mortality or specifically that Christ is the balm of our physical wounds. But myrrh is even more fascinating than that. Myrrh has received some negative attention lately. Many people think of it as unsafe because the more we analyze it, the more it starts to look kind of scary. Myrrh contains furanoid compounds, more than any other oils. Furanoid compounds are phototoxic -they cause sunburns. Myrrh contains phenols and ketones considered unsafe by biochemists. Myrrh contains acetic and formic acid -bee stings and ant bites. It also contains xylene, which can be found at your local toxic waste dump. The fact is; when broken down into its parts it contains danger, pain, suffering, and struggles -- much like our lives.

But the miracle is this! When blended by God, when left in its natural state, when the finger print of God is left upon it, all these scary chemicals interact perfectly together to render myrrh one of the most mild oils you can put on your body and one of the most healing. So much so, that for thousands of years the Egyptians used myrrh as a sunscreen, just as we do today with our pure therapeutic grade oils.

The lesson myrrh teaches us is that although life is full of struggles, pain, and danger; if we allow the fingerprint of God to be upon our lives, He will use it to heal us instead.

Matthew 11:30 (NIV)

"For my yoke is easy and my burden is light."

The wise men knew much of our Savior. In reality the gifts given to Christ represented His entire mission. They teach us that He will be wounded for our transgressions, that he will heal us both physically and spiritually. Gold represents our heritage and that of Christ, the Son of God.

Romans 8:17 (NIV)

"Now if we are children, then we are heirs—heirs of God and co-heirs with Christ, if indeed we share in his sufferings in order that we may also share in his glory."

This Christmas season I hope we can remember the message the wise men gave and allow Gods fingerprint to be upon all of our lives. Essential oils are a gift, but they are not the only gift. Life is full of blessings that make all the struggles worth it." (end of article)

----

dōTERRA Certified Pure Therapeutic Grade® essential oils represent the safest, purest, and most beneficial essential oils available today. They are gently and skillfully distilled from plants that have been patiently harvested at the perfect moment by experienced growers from around the world for ideal extract composition and efficacy. Experienced essential oil users will immediately recognize dōTERRA's superior quality standard for naturally safe, purely effective therapeutic-grade essential oils.

A few years back my husband, Evan, was hired by a private laboratory to build a piece of equipment for extracting essential oils from the Kava Kava plant. The process used chemicals to extract the oils and when it was condensed down into a highly potent substance, it still contained the chemical and was not entirely pure. Now he and I understand why this purity is critical. Because chemical extraction is not the exception, rather the more common practice, we must use care when selecting our oils.

Basic and Common Uses of Essential Oils

(fromhttp://www.sharedoterra.com/wp-content/uploads/2009/09/Essential+oil+concerns&+symptomatic+usage.pdf)

Essential oils are natural, safe, and therefore can be used freely. However, please note a few cautions:

1. NEVER PUT ANY ESSENTIAL OIL DIRECTLY IN THE EAR OR EYE. If any oil ever does get in these areas, dilute with a fractionated coconut oil, olive, or vegetable oil.

2. If any oil is ever too strong, or causes any type of irritation, you can dilute with one of the above oils and this will immediately alleviate any discomfort. Do not dilute with water. If an oil has gotten too close to my eyes, I will just put a couple of drops of coconut or olive oil on my finger and run it across my eyelid and this helps.

3. Remember you only need a couple of drops of the oil for each application. Also, unlike traditional over the counter drugs, you can apply these more often. It is better to apply a little more often, than a lot at one time.

Here are some examples of common ailments and the essential oils that can have a beneficial effect.

- ACNE: Melaleuca (alternafolia), geranium, lavender

- ALLERGIES: Lavender, Purify Blend; Respiratory Blend (Breathe); apply to sole of the foot, or put on palms of hands and cup hands and inhale; A drop or two under the nose can also help. (I would diffuse regularly to help reduce allergens in the air. I would diffuse Purify, Immune Blend, Breathe, or peppermint.)

- ANXIETY/DEPRESSION: Serenity, Balance, ylang ylang, sandalwood, frankincense, Citrus Bliss; I would put this under my nose, on the back of my neck or on my chest, or somewhere where I could smell it throughout the day. I would also diffuse one of these oils regularly.

- ASTHMA: Respiratory Blend (Breathe), wintergreen, Eucalyptus (Radiata), lemon, lavender, frankincense, marjoram; Rub on soles of feet 2-3 times daily, also rub on chest. Also, I would diffuse the oils daily to possibly reduce any airborne asthma triggers. (I would diffuse Purify, Immune Blend, peppermint or Eucalyptus (Radiata))

- BEE STINGS, BUG BITES: Purify, lavender

- BLISTERS: Melaleuca (alternafolia), lavender, sandalwood, frankincense

- BURNS: Lavender

- SUNBURN: Lavender; peppermint can also be cooling for a sunburn

- COLD SORES/CANKER SORES: On Guard(r) , lavender or sandalwood
- COLDS: On Guard(r), peppermint, Melaleuca (alternafolia), eucalyptus, lemon; apply to chest and spine. You can also apply a warm compress to help the oils penetrate deeper.
- COUGH: Breathe, Eucalyptus (Radiata), eucalyptus w/peppermint, eucalyptus w/ Lemon
- CROUP: Breathe, Eucalyptus (Radiata); Apply to chest and along spine
- EAR INFECTIONS: Melaleuca (alternafolia) w/ lavender on cotton ball and put in ear over night. I also put some around the ear area, but remember never in the ear. You can also use the Immune Blend or thyme.
- FATIGUE: May help to apply Elevate or peppermint behind neck or on feet
- INSECT BITES/BEE STINGS: (non-toxic bug repellant) Purify blend would be my first choice, also try geranium, lavender, cinnamon, rosemary, basil, thyme, peppermint—most give short lasting protection, usually less than 2 hours, so reapply),
- PINK EYE: Melaleuca (alternafolia), lavender; Apply to area around the eye. Be careful not to get in the eye or too close to the eye.

- RSV: Rub the Breathe or eucalyptus on the chest area, and also on the spine. If needed, you can dilute. You can also mix the eucalyptus with peppermint or lemon.

- RUNNY NOSE OR CONGESTION: Breathe or eucalyptus on sides of nose—eyes may water when you do this, so either close your eyes for a few minutes, or dilute with coconut oil.

- SORE THROAT: Gargle with oregano and lemon. Put a couple drops of each in an ounce or two of water, and gargle as long as you can stand it. (I warn you this is nasty, but one time has usually been enough to take care of it for me, also you may want to have the coconut or vegetable oil handy in case any of it gets on your lips, it may burn a bit.) You can also gargle with the Immune Blend. Breathe, the respiratory blend is also good for throat viruses, and you can apply this directly to the throat, for your kids who cannot do the nasty tasting things.

- STREP THROAT: Put a couple of drops of the Immune Blend in some water and drink the water, or gargle with oregano and lemon; Oregano, frankincense, myrrh; rub on throat, chest and back of neck.

- TENSION HEADACHE: Apply Past Tense®, peppermint or wintergreen on temples, around hairline, across the forehead, and on the back of the neck, can also apply it to soles of feet.

- SINUS HEADACHE: Breathe, Eucalyptus (Radiata), peppermint; Apply across forehead and around sinus area.
- SORE MUSCLES: Apply peppermint or Serenity on affected muscles.
- STOMACH/DIGESTION: Peppermint or Digest Zen blend. Rub this on stomach area. For smaller children, you may want to dilute it with a carrier oil. Ginger is also a good one for stomach problems.
- DIARRHEA: Rub peppermint or Digest Zen on the stomach.
- CONSTIPATION: Rub peppermint or Digest Zen on the stomach. You can also try ginger.
- HEARTBURN: Digest Zen, peppermint, lemon, ginger, anise; Put a couple drops in a capsule; Can also add a couple drops of lemon to 8 oz of water. By ingesting lemon juice and/or essential oils, the stomach stops excreting digestive acids, therefore alleviating heartburn or other stomach ailments.
- NAUSEA: Rubbing a couple of drops of peppermint behind the ears may help.
- MOLD: Diffuse some Purify Blend or Immune Blend
- PAIN: Deep Blue, wintergreen, peppermint, white fir

- SCRAPES, CUTS AND BRUISES: Lavender,
- STRESS: Lavender, orange, ylang ylang, lemon, Serenity; diffuse or apply somewhere where you can smell it throughout the day—i.e. back of neck, under nose, on chest.

Properties of Single Oils

- ANALGESIC/ANESTHETIC: Clove, Ginger, Lavender, Myrrh, Wintergreen
- ANTISEPTIC: Thyme, clove, oregano, Melaleuca (alternafolia), eucalyptus radiate, cassia, Lavender & Lemon
- ANTIBACTERIAL: Basil, Cassia, Cinnamon, Eucalyptus (Radiata), Geranium, Lemongrass, Marjoram, Oregano, Peppermint, Rosemary & Melaleuca (alternafolia)
- ANTI COAGULANT: Cassia, Cinnamon, Clove, Ginger , Helichrysum & Wintergreen
- ANTI-INFLAMMATORY: Basil, Cassia, Cinnamon, Clove, Eucalyptus (Radiata), Frankincense, Geranium, Ginger, Lavender, Lemongrass, Myrrh, Oregano, Peppermint, Melaleuca (alternafolia), Wintergreen, & Ylang ylang
- ANTI-FUNGAL Cassia, Cinnamon, Clove, White Fir, Geranium, Lavender, Lemongrass, Marjoram, Oregano, Peppermint, Rosemary, Melaleuca (alternafolia) & Thyme

- ANTI-INFECTIOUS: Cypress
- ANTI-OXIDANT: Clove, White Fir, Geranium & Myrrh
- ANTI-PARASITIC: Basil, Cinnamon, Clove, Lemongrass, Myrrh, Oregano, Peppermint, Rosemary, Melaleuca (alternafolia), Thyme, & Ylang ylang
- ANTIVIRAL: Basil, Cassia, Cinnamon, Clove, Eucalyptus (Radiata), Myrrh, Oregano, Peppermint, Sandalwood, Melaleuca (alternafolia) & Thyme
- ANTI SPASMODIC: Basil, Cypress, Geranium, Wintergreen, & Ylang ylang
- CIRCULATORY STIMULANT: Cinnamon & Cypress & Helichrysum
- EXPECTORANT: Cypress, Eucalyptus (Radiata), Frankincense, Ginger, Lemon, & Marjoram

The Science

Antiviral and Antimicrobial Properties of Essential Oils, by Dominique Baudoux (Excerpts)

During the 1960s, Dr. Jean Valnet gave rise to the rebirth of aromatherapy, which split up into several schools, allowing thousands of doctors to get familiar with an anti-infectious technique not acknowledged by medical schools. Encouraged by hundreds of thousands of patients, a wide-ranging movement was born.

Anti-Infectious Properties

Antibacterial

This is the most widely studied area of essential oils; this property is the only one that is really well-known and used regularly. In fact, many people associate 'aromatherapy' with 'anti-infectious therapy'.

The capacity of essential oils to neutralize germs is now irrefutable. Experimental studies were undertaken in France by Chamberland as early as 1887. In 1888, Cadeac and Meunier published the results of their own research (Annales de l'Institut Pasteur). Many in-vitro confirmations were performed by pharmacists and doctors; results were conclusive. In his book, Antiseptiques Essentiels, published in 1938, René-Maurice Gattefosse described the already considerable advancement of the research.

Molecules with the highest anti-bacterial coefficient are: carvacrol, thymol and eugenol; all three are phenols. Not a phenol (but related, with a benzenic core), cinnamic aldehyde has an anti-infectious activity comparable to phenols. Thanks to these four molecules, any aromatherapy-savvy practitioner will be able to master most common infections.

Alcohols with ten carbon atoms (or monoterpenols) come immediately after: geraniol, linalool, thujanol and myrcenol, terpineol, menthol and piperitol are the most well-known. Reliable, broad-spectrum molecules, they are useful in numerous cases of bacterial infections. Aldehydes are also somewhat antibacterial; the most widely used are neral and geranial (citrals), citronnellal and cuminal.

Ketones are interesting for the treatment of mucupurulent infectious states (usually a strictly indirect action): verbenone, thujone, borneone (camphor), pinocamphone, cryptone, fenchone, menthone, piperitone and carvone.

Anti-Fungal

Fungal infections are a hot topic today, due to the overuse and abuse of antibiotics by most members of the medical profession; as we all know, antibiotics are first and foremost microscopic fungi. The molecular groups with the strongest antibacterial action are also active on fungi. However, treatment must be over a longer period. Fundamental studies have also revealed the anti-fungal activity of alcohols and sesquiterpenic lactones.

Antiviral

The mad parasites of any and all forms of life, viruses give rise to pro-teiform pathologies, some of which medical science can do nothing to cure. Classic responses to these infections are very limited, so essential oils are a godsend in treating viral problems, from the most common to the most fearsome.

Molecules from many chemical families have shown an in-vitro antiviral activity, among them monoterpenols and monoterpenals. Ketones, and especially rare cryptone, have shown an interesting capacity to fight naked viruses. Aldehydes, whether used internally or in the atmosphere, are good complementary treatments for patients with viral infections.

Generally, viruses are highly sensitive to aromatic molecules, and some severe viral pathologies may show a vast improvement following their use. A fact of the highest interest, unearthed during fundamental research and clinical experiments: normal cells of patients under aromatic treatment seem to acquire a special resistance to viral penetration. (end of article)

Antibiotics vs. Therapeutic-Grade Essential Oils

by Joan Barice, M.D. (excerpts)

Speaking as a medical doctor, all physicians are aware of the increasing problem of resistance of bacteria to antibiotics. This is especially a problem with bacteria which cause life threatening infections. It is a result of overusing antibiotics, and of using them when they are not appropriate.

Overusing antibacterial soaps may also contribute to the problem. Prevention is best, of course.

Allowing natural immunity to work when infections are self-limiting or not likely to cause serious consequences is also important, as is not treating viruses with antibiotics which will not work anyway.

Essential oils can be very effective in treating many bacterial, viral and other infections, without causing resistance. The natural variation in the chemical constituents in whole plants depending on climate, altitude, and other factors protects against this resistance, as do the many chemical constituents in whole oils as opposed to using one isolated "active" ingredient.

The problem is, most doctors are not trained in using oils, but are well trained in using potent antibiotics. If you are trying to enlighten a doctor, who generally has had no training on essential oils, I would suggest providing scientific references that give the available evidence of the effectiveness of essential oils in treating infections.

Examples of published articles on essential oil research, especially those in medical journals:

- Dr. Kurt Schnaubelt's book "Medical Aromatherapy" has a list of some basic research, including the following:
- 1960: Maruzella demonstrated antibacterial and antifungal effects of hundreds of aromatic compounds
- 1987: Deininger and Lembke demonstrated antiviral activity of essential oils and their isolated components
- 1973: Wagner and Sprinkmeyer in 1973 did research on a 170 year old blend of distilled oils still available in Germany. The effects of melissa and the other oils in Kosterfrau Melissengeist had been empirically known since Paracelsus (about 1500). They concluded that, with varying degrees of intensity, there was an inhibiting influence on all the bacteria tested, (Pneumococcus, Klebsiella pneumoniae, Staphlococcus aureus haemolyticus, Neisseria catarrhalis, Streptococcus haemolyticus,
- Proteus vulgaris, Hemophilus influenza, Haemophilus pertussis, Candida albicans, Escherichia coli-

- Aerobacter group, various Corynnebacteria, and Listeria) and stated the large spectrum of this inhibitory action is as broad as or even greater than that of wide-spectrum antibiotics.
- Schnaubelt lists even earlier basic science research showing it has been known a long time that essential oils have antimicrobial effects:
- 1800-2002: Numerous animal and in vitro studies - evidence that all essential oils are antiseptic, some more than others and that many are effective against certain fungi, bacteria and viruses.
- 1881: Koch demonstrated the bactericidal action of essence of turpentine against anthrax spores
- 1887: Chamberland demonstrated bactericidal activity of essences of oregano, cinnamon and clove on bacillus anthracis1910: Martindale showed essential oil of oregano is the strongest plant-derived antiseptic known to date, 25 to 76 times more active than phenol on colobacillus.

WEB RESOURCES

Essential oil uses, protocols and testimonials:
www.everythingessential.me

Resource of essential oil videos and their applications:
www.youtube.com

Every essential oil practitioner needs this book: ***Modern Essentials: A Contemporary Guide to the Therapeutic Use of Essential Oils.*** Find it at: http://essentialoilsbook.com/

Membership, Discounts and Products:
www.healedbyoils.com and www.beautifuldoterra.com

Chapter 8: Coaching Basics

Leelo Bush, Ph.D.

As you are implementing the tips in this book, you likely feel better and more vibrant already. By adding the coaching component, you can easily learn to help others as well. In this chapter, we'll explore life coaching, Christian life coaching and wellness coaching specifically.

Coaching presupposes a deliberately formed, confidential relationship for the purpose of improving one or more areas of a person's life.

There are three criteria required for the coaching process to be successful.

1. **First**, there must be one or more areas of someone's life that they want to improve.

2. **Second,** the person must be willing to allow someone else, such as the coach, into the process.

It is your job as the coach, to determine whether someone is coachable or not.

3. **Third,** the person has to be agreeable to make some changes, meaning the person being coached will have to think and behave differently than in the past. We all

know that if we keep doing what we are doing, we will keep getting the same result

If you were to eliminate even one of the above criteria, it would not be possible to have a successful coaching relationship. It is your job as the coach, to determine whether someone is coachable or not. Just because someone says they want coaching does not mean that this arrangement will necessarily be fruitful or beneficial.

Characteristics of Coachable Clients and Situations

- The desired outcome must be in line with the word of God.
- The timing must be led by the Holy Spirit. In other words, both the coach and client must feel secure that now is the time to proceed.
- The client must have control over the desired actions and options. The client needs to be in a place to be able to speak freely and confidently with the coach.
- The client is able to accurately describe the situation and how their actions might affect it.
- The client is willing to risk doing things differently in order to achieve the change.

- The change must be measurable in some way that can be communicated to the coach.

Characteristics of an Uncoachable Client or Situation

- The client does not have control over the desired actions. For example, the client's superior will not allow a change in how things are done.
- The client is unable or unwilling to be truthful about the situation.
- The client is frightened about making a change sufficiently to paralyze progress.
- The client lacks a high level of interest in seeing change occur.
- The client thinks no action taken will make a difference in the outcome (fatalism).
- The client primarily wants to complain about the situation without taking any action or responsibility for the outcome.
- The client lacks follow through to make agreed-upon changes.
- The client is not willing to take a close look at the situation and/or options.
- The actions required must be taken by someone other than the client. For example, if a woman is seeking

coaching about something her husband needs to do, coaching the wife will not be affective. Instead, it is best the husband partner in the coaching relationship.

Advice Giving Versus Coaching

Some people are drawn to life coaching because they have been sought out for sharing sound-advice and they enjoy providing this kind of support. However, advice giving and speaking from experience are more akin to mentoring than coaching. Coaching means partnering with another, rather than telling them what to do.

In order to be an effective coach, you need to learn to ask the right questions. This will help the people you are coaching discover their own solutions. When people own their solutions, they are three times more likely to take action on them.

Your questions need to be simple, direct and allow for open-ended answers. Their purpose is to stimulate creative thinking and reflection, as well as enable disclosure of pertinent details. Here are some great questions to ask.

- What outcome do you want?
- How does this line up with what you believe God wants you to do?
- What is getting in your way?

- What is the cost to the delay?
- What are other ways to think about your challenge(s)?
- What is the most significant action you could take right now?
- What new systems or skills will support your progress?

It is very important to focus on the client's responses. Some people make the mistake of planning their follow-up question prior to hearing everything their client says. Can you see how this might present a barrier to effective coaching?

The coach needs to be genuinely caring and curious. Listen closely to *everything* your client says before asking a follow-up question. You may think that you have an inkling about what is going on, but it is always best to allow the client to confirm it.

Some Great ways to Ask Follow-up Questions

- Ask for clarification: "Tell me more." "Would you elaborate on that?"
- Ask for client's interpretation of events: "What does this mean to you?" "What else might it mean?" Ask for 3-5 more possible meanings.
- Ask for the next level or for a bigger game: "How can you take it up a notch?"

- "What is the next step?"
- "Is it manageable or does it need to be broken down into smaller steps?"
- Ask for the client to gauge their level of commitment: "Rate your level of commitment on a scale of 1-10 with ten

Coaching means partnering with another, rather than telling them what to do. You help your client gain clarity and aid them in processing their thoughts to arrive at the best decisions.

being the greatest, that you will take action?" If their response is not a 9 or 10, ask: "What would increase your commitment to taking the agreed-upon action?"
- When you receive a report on the results, ask the client: "How does that feel?"
- "How it might be different if you lean into the situation rather than trying to ignore or avoid it?"

Can you see how these are questions that will get your client thinking about options and actions they can take? If at some point in your coaching session, you feel an urgency to interject either personal experience or revelation, ask your client's permission to do so first.

You could say something like this. "I just had another thought about this. May I have your permission to share?" Almost always, your client will agree. Then it is safe for you to proceed. Remember, this is your client's coaching session. All focus must be on your client and their needs, at all times.

You may find in someone's coaching sessions that you keep revisiting the same issue time and time again. If this is the case, there may come a time when you feel led to say something difficult or tough to your client. It is best you know right now, not all coaching produces feel-good moments. There are times your client may have to face down some difficult challenges. This is a good thing and as it should be. If you are doing your job as a coach, you are partnering with your client to come up to a higher level and providing a safe space to do so.

Always love and help your clients understand they are in a safe place to process, share and challenge themselves candidly. Most of the time, the best way to get beyond a challenge or difficulty is to go through it. Your client will appreciate the breakthrough, even if it is uncomfortable for a time.

Remember, duty is yours to coach them. The results and timing are up to God. You are not the author of the results, so do not let it upset you if you are not seeing the results you think should be there. It could be the client is not ready. It might be that the step was too large to take and needs to be broken down.

However, if you find over time that your client is not taking agreed-upon actions, you will have to assess whether now is a good time for them to be involved with coaching. It could be that your client needs to work out some other things before moving successfully into the coaching process.

There are cases, from time to time, when you may need to refer someone for counseling. If you feel this way, please be honest with your client and tell them that you suspect based on your experience and training, that you may not be the best person to help them. However, you will do what you can to refer them to someone better equipped to assist them.

This is where it will be really helpful for you to have some resources in your community. Make sure you get out, do some networking, and meet other service providers in your area. This will benefit you in two ways. It will introduce you to possible referral sources for your clients and it will also acquaint your community with the service you provide so that if needed, they can refer clients to you as well.

Some Special Tips for Christian Coaches

- I recommend you pray prior to every session. Depending upon your clients' receptivity, you may want to pray by yourself before the session or with your client.

- Become knowledgeable about scripture related to health and wellness as well as God's promises in His Word. You will find many of them throughout this book. Read and reread this information. Commit it to memory.

- I highly recommend you also take the Certified Christian Life Coach program (CLCC) that we offer. (http://www.pccca.org/cclc_teleclass.html) It will give you so much more depth of knowledge in the coaching profession to be able to help more people in different ways. You will also learn the F-L-O-W coaching model. In this training I also go into depth about the 10 Christian coaching proficiencies, along with scripture references.

In the CCLC, I also teach:

- Coaching Systems, Methods, or Models
- Values-Based Life Design
- Purposeful Passion and Finding Yours
- Developing Clear Vision and Mission Statements

- Dealing with Change
- Overcoming Obstacles
- Necessary Listening Skills
- Two Distinct Anatomies (detailed procedures) for Coaching Sessions
- Practical Business Procedures and Operations
- Ethics, Accountability, Liability and Best Practices
- Business, Marketing, Branding, and Much More

10 Christian Coaching Proficiencies© in the order they are presented

The **10 Christian Coaching Proficiencies**© make up the process by which we coach from a truly Biblical foundation. These scripture(s) and discussions on implementation can be found in the CCLC training.

1. Inspire anointed conversation.

2. Encourage awareness of God's plan.

3. Draw out excellence; let success happen.

4. Demonstrate love and grace toward the client.

5. Optimize and celebrate the client's efforts.

6. Do not presume you know. Ask, and then listen.

7. Abate fear with confidence in God's divine purpose.

8. Pray for discernment about priorities.

9. Improve communication skills.

10. Build supportive environments.

Our goal as Christian coaches is to help clients develop to the point where making the right choices and responding, as opposed to reacting, comes naturally because they are seeking the Lord before any other thing. (Ref. Matthew 6:33)

Coaching will help your client become more disciplined in life. We want clients to develop good habits. We know it is a lot easier for clients to accomplish goals, when action steps become second nature.

Here are some supportive environments that you may wish to suggest for your clients.

- Regular Devotional Time
- Church Family
- Knowledge of God's Word
- Christian Fellowship
- Family and Friends
- Daily Spiritual Disciplines
- Other _____

I challenge you to coach fearlessly, from a position of faith. We must love our clients more than our perceived self-image. God's Word tells us that perfect love casts out all fear.

1 John 4:18 (NIV)

"There is no fear in love. But perfect love drives out fear, because fear has to do with punishment. The one who fears is not made perfect in love."

Wellness Coaching Specifics

Similar to what we have talked about previously, a wellness coach does not give advice; rather the wellness coach collaborates with the person they are coaching to help him or her create processes and systems by using the following steps:

- First the coach and client identify strengths and weaknesses. An easy way to do this is to use the Wellness Coaching Circle Model© included in the appendix.
- Then the coach and client together consider an area where the client desires most to make a positive change.
- To do so, the coach and client explore various options. They may discuss the history at how the client arrived at their situation today. They may review challenges. And as they discuss possibilities, they also look for support systems.

- Together the coach and client set up specific, measurable, attainable, realistic, and time -specific goals. This is also referred to as the SMART goal setting system.

An important aspect to wellness coaching is the accountability piece. It is crucial that the client remains accountable to taking the agreed-upon steps so that their goals can be met. Initially the client learns to be accountable to the coach. But then, it is the coach's job to help the client become self-accountable. What we are really doing with coaching is rather than giving a man a fish, we teach a man to fish. Your goal is to work yourself out of a job, as less and less support is needed over time rather than create greater dependence on the coaching. As your client achieves their goals, their satisfaction will increase creating word-of-mouth referrals for you.

With coaching, wellness coaching specifically, we work with the client to create on-going, sustainable behaviors that will result in a healthy lifestyle with wellness as the result.

As a wellness coach, you bring several things to this coaching relationship.

- You bring your training and experience.
- You bring your communication skills.
- You bring your ability to help the client create steps that will result in behavior modification.

Wellness coaching can be done entirely in person. Many people prefer that. However, today coaching by phone or by e-mail is almost equally as effective and far more time-efficient. Coaching over the phone or by email, removes all geographic barriers. Essentially you could be working with and coaching anyone located anywhere in the world with phone or Internet access.

Listen closely to everything your client says before asking a follow-up question.

Why would a person seek wellness coaching?

Perhaps they need to make some changes to build a better lifestyle. They may have a goal to quit a particular habit such as smoking. If this is something you have overcome, you might even consider making smoking cessation your coaching niche! Such a coach would possibly help their client explore various options to quit. They might include support groups, nicotine replacement, or even going "cold turkey", as they say. The smoking cessation coach would also explore challenges with their client. They would take a look at any previous efforts that had been made and the results achieved. From this history they would learn what has not worked and how similar approaches could be modified for greater effect.

Other reasons that someone might seek wellness coaching would be to increase their fitness level, make better nutrition choices, improve their knowledge about and create sustainable lifestyle habits to support on-going health conditions such as recovery from illness or injury, diabetes, high blood pressure, chronic pain, and so forth.

As a former home healthcare agency founder and operator, I witness how significantly this industry has changed. Among these changes, I have seen a dramatic increase in health and wellness coaching modalities added to home healthcare regimens.

In most cases, the healthcare provider (nurse, certified nursing assistant, therapist, etc.) is not present outside of visit times. It is left to the patient and their wellness coach to support them in any type of behavior modification that will help the client regain their health or sustain positive change.

A typical case might involve someone recovering from an accident or surgery where they need to continue to perform physical therapist-prescribed exercises in their home.

You can also find wellness coaches with training in alcohol or substance-abuse, who are able to specialize in this particular niche by combining their personal, life experiences having lived with such disorders with formal wellness coach training. This will bring the benefit of the coach's skills, experience and empathy to their coaching client.

To give our wellness coaches a place to begin their coaching session, I have created the Wellness Coaching Circle Model©. You will find a larger version of this exercise in your appendix.

To use this model, have the person you are coaching grade their level of wellness in each of the 10 categories. They will rate each category with 10 (ten) being the highest or ideal wellness and 1 (one) indicating extreme difficulty. As they do this, have them place a dot in the center of the section in the space corresponding to the wellness number. Then connect the dots to create a visual display of how the client sees their levels of wellness in each area. This will reveal an overview of needs as well as help to identify the most urgent areas to be addressed.

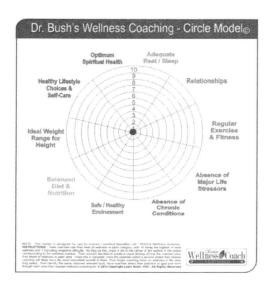

Once this is complete, have your client select a section where they believe coaching will most likely have the greatest *immediate* benefit to them. Then begin coaching them on wellness in this particular area asking key questions to identify what they see the issue being and how they would like to approach it. To best do this, first identify the issue, then discover relevant facts, then have them select their direction or goals and work through each area for which they request wellness coaching. .

When coaching someone, it is fairly typical, to discover issues in other areas as well in which coaching could be beneficial. If you are not familiar or qualified with these other areas, you will need to refer your client. However, if you intend to make this your profession it is incumbent upon you to gain additional training or participate in continuing education programs in coaching as well as specific coaching specialties.

A Note About Professional Liability Insurance

Students of Beautiful Life International / PCCCA are eligible for professional liability and health insurance through our provider, at very affordable rates. You will find a link to the insurance center from our resources page. If you need assistance with this, please contact the Academy by emailing admin@pccca.org.

Free Gift For You!

Please go to
pammaldonado.com/free-gift
to download your
free gift!

To your amazing health and
happiness in body, mind and
spirit!
Pam Maldonado

Chapter 9: Putting it all Together

Congratulations on arriving at the final chapter. By now you have likely concluded that wellness is really all about life. To me, wellness coaching is helping people find balance in their lives. As Christian wellness coaches, we base our life balance on the inclusion of the Holy Spirit and the teachings of Jesus Christ. When we have balance in our body, mind, and spirit, life is good!

A client may come to you for weight loss and as you are meeting with them, you may just find out that the reason they cannot lose the weight is because they just never get any sleep! It really can be as simple as that: fix the sleep, fix the weight! Wellness issues are so inter-twined and amazing. When one aspect is out of whack, another is affected. If things are not changed, the entire body suffers as well as the spirit, and disease soon takes over in one form or another.

Remember, wellness coaching is all about balance and lifestyle choices. Lifestyle choices are the answer to preventing the chronic disease epidemic. Wellness coaching is the obvious answer and a potentially lucrative field.

If you have been provoked by reading this book or participating in the webinars to do more research in the area most interesting to you, my goal has been accomplished. There is so much more to learn than what I have presented to you, but you will become an expert in the area that is specific to your interests. You have done the ground work and are ready to get started, creating your new you if you so choose.

If you enrolled and participated in the webinars, you have received many of the forms you will need to start your wellness practice. You are welcome to modify them to reflect your goals in order to suit your needs and those of your clients'.

Remember, coaching is client-driven. Your job is to ask stimulating questions to help your client identify solutions to challenges. More importantly, the work you do alongside your client is also Christ-centered. Invite the Holy Spirit to be present and expect Him to actively participate in the process. You will feel a "nudge" from Him as you coach to speak truth in love to your client. And, as Dr. Bush suggested previously, ask your client if you may share with them what you are sensing. Then, if your client is open, tell your client what you have been asked to share. I tell you, it is so amazing when this happens! When your clients are open to the Holy Spirit as well, it is not uncommon to learn that they too, were sensing the same thing! Both of you will just want to get up and do a dance of praise! It is hard to describe that feeling because sometimes as a coach you are wondering where the session is going; however, you keep moving forward in faith believing it is being directed in the right way. When something like that happens, it just solidifies the presence of the Holy Spirit, and you know you are not attempting this on your own. It is hard to describe, but so amazing! You will see!

Let us summarize and review what you actually have in your possession now that we have completed most of this book. If you are reading this in conjunction with the Christian Wellness Coach training and certification program, and printed out all of the materials I have made available to you, you should have a nice collection to get you well on your way as a Christian wellness coach, if that is your goal. If you intend to use them to develop your own, personal wellness plan, that is fine too. Should you opt to become a Certified Christian Wellness Coach, you will now have personal experience, training and the credentials to confidently help others in this profession.

Let us review exactly what resources you will have.

We have covered three main categories of wellness: body, mind, and spirit. Everything else stems from these three including:

Exercise	Weight Control
Nutrition	Sleep
Medical	Financial
Social/Emotional	Vocational
Relationships	Stress

We have discussed and learned about the many passages in the Bible that give us straight advice on each topic, thus basing our program on Biblical truths. Those of you who completed the "Talk with God" assignment in the course have spent time with God seeking His guidance and direction so we can do what we are called to do. Therefore our plan in essence, is God's plan for our lives.

We have learned how to assess our or our client's wellness and how to set goals. An extensive wellness journal (included in the training component) is a tool for those who wish to track their accomplishments.

We have introduced a bit of humor to keep a light, positive attitude toward life. We have included prayers and scripture to keep reassuring us we are doing the right thing. We discovered our secret desires about our eating habits and gained awareness about them, resulting in greater understanding of ourselves making us better able to help our clients understand themselves.

We learned about our relationships with food and how to change our thinking over to God's way of thinking.

We acquired tools and knowledge to change our thinking about anything so we can do the right things as a living example of Godly character. Negative thinking will no longer control us as we learned not only how to change our thinking, but how to use affirmations and changing negative thoughts into positive affirmations.

We have contracts for weight loss and accountability. We have exercise charts and other tools to help with creating exercise programs and goals to use with anyone. We have nutrition guidelines that are easy and adaptable for anyone.

The journal for tracking and creating awareness about eating and exercise throughout the days and weeks will be invaluable to your clients.

We now have new tools to help you understand, increase awareness of, and deal with stress we all experience.

We now have an understanding of the importance of sleep, and how sleep deprivation affects our overall quality of living and immune system.

We now know the many healing qualities of natural health that are available to us and how to receive it.

We now better understand how relationships can harm or enhance our quality of life and productivity, and we have the tools to help our clients in this area of concern.

And finally, if you are taking the Wellness Coaching Course, you should have completed an activity that specifically spelled out your unique coaching plan and how it will be implemented. You were created by God for God, and your individual perspective in helping mankind, the crown of God's creation, will honor Him.

As a result of learning these concepts, you now possess an understanding that will give you confidence as you move forward. If you coach others, you will notice how unique each person's journey to wellness is. It reflects who God has created you to be and it will serve those people whom God has put into your path. It is up to you to use this gift in the way God has intended.

If this is God's plan, there is no stopping you if you are willing to do the work and never give up. You know you will come up against many roadblocks. Our adversary will want to keep you quiet! You are a threat! You must see through that and carry on with what God has equipped you to do! The need for wellness coaching is incredible as the health of our world's inhabitants is deteriorating by the minute! You are in great demand because:

- 7 out of 10 deaths each year among Americans are from chronic illnesses.
- Heart disease, cancer, and stroke account for more than 50% of all deaths each year!
- 75% of the $2.8 trillion in health care costs are due to chronic diseases!
- Many of these diseases and costs can be prevented by making lifestyle changes.
- Lifestyle change is what a Christian wellness coach facilitates.

Remember, wellness coaching is all about balance and lifestyle choices. Lifestyle choices are the answer to preventing the chronic disease epidemic. Wellness coaching is the obvious answer and a potentially lucrative field. By adding the spiritual component to the wellness profession, the success rates of your clients increase exponentially.

Now is the Time to Think about Your Wellness Coaching Niche

Many employers, health plans, and hospitals hire wellness coaches to improve the health and ultimately productivity of their employees. Large companies like Nike and Land's End hire wellness coaches, as do smaller companies. You just need to search and you will find many possibilities.

How Much Can a Wellness Coach Earn?

"Based on our discussions with hundreds of coaches in many settings, wellness coaches typically earn from $25 to $100 per coaching hour, or $50,000 to $100,000 a year, depending on the setting" according to Marci Alboher in an article, _Hot New Career: Wellness Coaching_.

Your earning potential can vary depending on what else you do with your coaching talent. Many coaches work in private practices. Others are also speaking, writing, conducting group classes, community projects, ethnic-related programs, therapy, personal training, and more. The possibilities are endless when you take your interests and strengths and create a wellness program of your own.

Based on our discussions with hundreds of coaches in many settings, wellness coaches typically earn from $25 to $100 per coaching hour, or $50,000 to $100,000 a year, depending on the setting"

For example, do you have a passion for eating and preparing healthy, natural, home-grown food? Is that your passion? What a help you could be to those who need that guidance. Have you overcome a wellness-related issue that others might benefit

210

God led you here for a purpose. He has equipped you with a plan, tools, and a need. People are crying out for help. You are now positioned to help them stay healthy resulting in more productive and fulfilling lives.

from as a result of your experience? Could you create a coaching niche based around that topic? Have you gone through a lot of loss in your life and you have learned how to live with joy in spite of it? Perhaps you would be able to work with others as they face loss, as well. Take your love, passion, and strengths and build your coaching practice around it. As I said, there is no end to what you can do and with the additional training available, you can enhance your credibility significantly.

There is far more to wellness than what we have covered here in this course. It is very important that you keep educating yourself on the many aspects of wellness in order to keep your own life in balance as well as those you may be coaching. I suggest you check out the various high-quality Christian coaching courses offered by the Professional Christian Coaching and Counseling Academy (www.pccca.org). There are so many options for strengthening your coaching skills. I will be offering more in depth courses that will enhance your learning from this introductory program. My goal is to help you take what you already know and help you specialize in the wellness area of greatest interest to you. I will also be offering one-on-one coaching to help you as well. Please subscribe to my newsletter to receive updates as to when these will be available along with new tips and news about this amazing and growing field. http://pammaldonado.com/free5

God led you here for a purpose. He has now equipped you with a plan, tools, and a need. People are crying out for help. You are now positioned to help them stay healthy resulting in more productive and fulfilling lives. It is now up to you to take the next step. How will you use this talent? Will you bury your talent, or will you invest it and multiply it tenfold like that parable of the talents (Matthew 25:14-30)?

Where are you going to make a difference in the world?

Where is God leading you? Who will you serve? Who will you help? How will you do this? How will you use and invest your knowledge that you now possess?

By now you know I am a huge fan of Dr. Don Colbert. His words resonate with me.

"Your health is up to you, and it is time to get serious. The clock is ticking, and there is urgency in the world today."

Pray about your new ministry. Expect big things! Do not limit God to being a small God. He does things in big ways! Expect it! Trust Him!

Appendix

Components of Christian Wellness

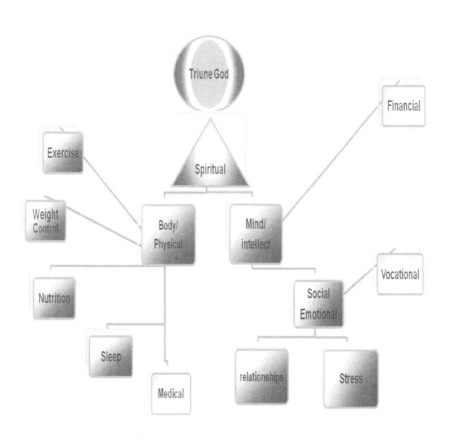

Weight Loss Chart

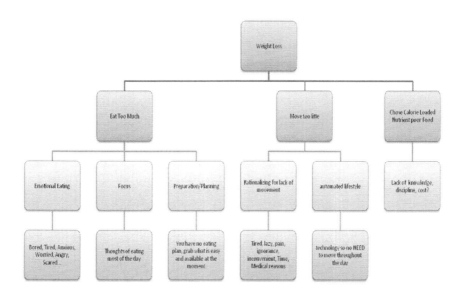

Center for Disease Control Exercise Plan

There are a lot of ways to get the physical activity you need!

If you're thinking, "How can I meet the Guidelines each week?" don't worry. You'll be surprised by the variety of activities you have to choose from. Basically anything counts, as long as it's at a moderate- or vigorous-intensity for at least 10 minutes at a time. If you're not sure where to start, here are some examples of weekly activity routines you may want to try.

Moderate Aerobic Activity Routines

	Monday	Tuesday	Wednesday	Thursday	Friday	Saturday	Sunday	Physical Activity TOTAL
Example 1	30 minutes of brisk walking	30 minutes of brisk walking	Resistance band exercises	30 minutes of brisk walking	30 minutes of brisk walking	Resistance band exercises	30 minutes of brisk walking	150 minutes moderate-intensity aerobic activity AND 2 days muscle strengthening
Example 2	30 minutes of brisk walking	60 minutes of playing softball	30 minutes of brisk walking	30 minutes of mowing the lawn		Heavy gardening	Heavy gardening	150 minutes moderate-intensity aerobic activity AND 2 days muscle strengthening

Vigorous Aerobic Activity Routines

	Monday	Tuesday	Wednesday	Thursday	Friday	Saturday	Sunday	Physical Activity TOTAL
Example 3	25 minutes of jogging	Weight lifting	25 minutes of jogging	Weight lifting	25 minutes of jogging			75 minutes vigorous-intensity aerobic activity AND 2 days muscle strengthening
Example 4	25 minutes of swimming laps		25 minutes of running	Weight training	25 minutes of singles tennis	Weight training		75 minutes vigorous-intensity aerobic activity AND 2 days muscle strengthening

Mix of Moderate and Vigorous Aerobic Activity Routines

	Monday	Tuesday	Wednesday	Thursday	Friday	Saturday	Sunday	Physical Activity TOTAL
Example 5	30 minutes of water aerobics / Weight lifting	30 minutes of jogging	30 minutes of brisk walking / Yoga		30 minutes of brisk walking	Yoga		90 minutes moderate-intensity aerobic activity AND 30 minutes vigorous-intensity aerobic activity AND 2 days muscle strengthening
Example 6	45 minutes of doubles tennis	Rock	climbing		30 minutes of vigorous hiking		45 minutes of doubles tennis	90 minutes moderate-intensity aerobic activity AND 30 minutes vigorous-intensity aerobic activity AND 2 days muscle strengthening

For more information, see www.cdc.gov/physicalactivity

What Are We Eating?

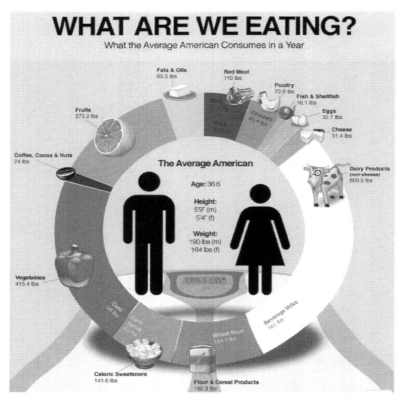

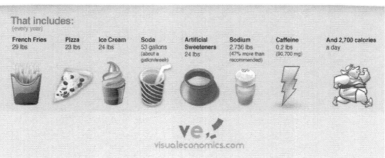

Dr. Bush's Wellness Coaching – Circle Model©

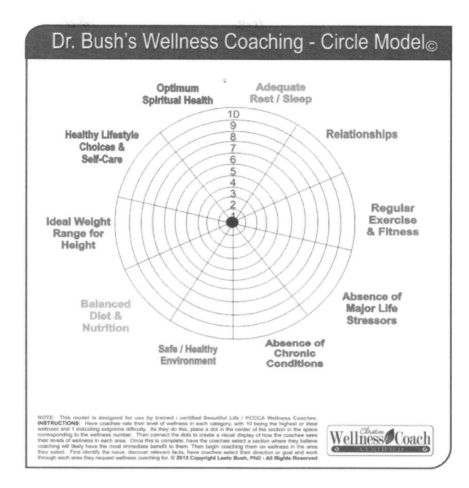

Signs of Stress

- Changes in Body
- Sweaty Palms
- Perspiring, Feeling Flushed
- Shortness of Breath
- Tight Neck and Shoulders
- Body tension
- Back Aches
- Muscle Twitching
- Jaw Pain
- Rapid Heartbeat
- Chest Pains
- Gastrointestinal Upset
- Dry Mouth
- Fatigue
- Poor Sleep
- Changes in Behavior
- Changes in Thinking
- Headaches
- High Blood Pressure
- Eye Strain
- Weight Loss or Gain
- Teeth Grinding
- Skin Rashes
- Increased Urination
- Frequent Colds/Flu
- Inattentiveness
- Mental Fatigue
- Inability to Focus
- Poor Concentration
- Forgetfulness
- Excessive worry
- Increased Negative Thinking
- Diminished Problem Solving Skills
- Difficulty Multi-Tasking
- Changes in Emotions
- Nervous
- Anxious
- Fearful
- Feeling on Edge
- Frustration
- Irritable
- Impatience
- Anger
- Disgusted
- Apathy
- Lack of Pleasure
- Sadness
- Discouraged
- Helpless
- Hopelessness
- Crying
- Lonely
- Depression
- Suspiciousness
- Dislike of Self
- Feeling Defensive
- Decreased Activity Level
- Lack of Enthusiasm
- Withdrawal from Social
- Relationships
- Rushing
- Increased Errors on the Job
- Argumentative, Defensive
- Uncooperative
- Overeating or Under eating
- Changes in Nicotine Use
- Misuse of Alcohol
- Drug Use
- Unsafe Driving
- Too Much or Not Enough Sleep

Index

abilities, 71
abnormalities, 102
abundance, 14, 135
academy, 4, 201, 211
accident, 199
accomplish, 73, 78, 82, 162, 195
accountability, 197, 207
activities, 20, 48, 51, 63, 68
addictions, 86
additives, 86
adrenaline, 106
adverse, 86, 90
aerobacter, 183
affective, 188
agency, 199
albicans, 182
alcohol, 125, 199
aldehyde, 178
allergens, 172
alternafolia, 171, 172, 173, 176, 177
alzheimer, 67
analgesic, 176
anesthetic, 176
anise, 175
anointed, 194
antacids, 48
anthrax, 183
antibacterial, 176
antibiotic, 158, 163, 179
antifungal, 182
antimicrobial, 183
antioxidants, 86, 92, 98
antiseptic, 173, 183
antiviral, 158, 180, 182
anxiety, 172

Free Gift For You!

Please go to
pammaldonado.com/free-gift
to download your
free gift!

To your amazing health and
happiness in body, mind and
spirit!
Pam Maldonado

Made in the USA
San Bernardino, CA
29 July 2014